Praise for *Target 100*

"When I was losing weight, Liz was more than my coach; she was my rock, and I couldn't have done it without her. She just got it, because she'd been through it herself (and helped about a million other people through it, too). *Target 100* is Liz in book form—smart, supportive, and full of practical, simple solutions. Liz changed my life and my whole concept of dieting— and now can change, yours too."

—JESSICA SIMPSON

"Liz is no joke. She helps people change their lives, me included. She is special and if you're ready for real change, you're ready for *Target 100*."

—CHARLES BARKLEY

"Liz Josefsberg gets it! For anyone who has struggled with weight loss, Liz connects the dots in a way that only someone who has been through it can. Add her expertise and experience on top of it and you have a real handbook for success."

—KATIE COURIC

"If you are struggling with your body, Liz has walked in your shoes and understands the practical steps for clever solutions."

—MEHMET OZ, MD, PROFESSOR AT NEW YORK-PRESBYTERIAN: COLUMBIA UNIVERSITY MEDICAL CENTER

"I just love the perspective that Liz brings to weight loss. Need a shot in the arm? Look no further than Liz Josefberg's *Target 100*. So many clients have benefited from Liz's exceptional guidance and simple approach, and you will, too."

—ROCCO DISPIRITO

Target 100

Target
100

THE WORLD'S SIMPLEST WEIGHT LOSS PROGRAM IN 6 EASY STEPS

LIZ JOSEFSBERG

BENBELLA

BenBella Books, Inc.
Dallas, TX

This book is for informational purposes only. It is not intended to serve as a substitute for professional medical advice. The author and publisher specifically disclaim any and all liability arising directly or indirectly from the use of any information contained in this book. A health-care professional should be consulted regarding your specific medical situation.

BenBella

BenBella Books, Inc.
10440 N. Central Expressway, Suite 800
Dallas, TX 75231
www.benbellabooks.com
Send feedback to feedback@benbellabooks.com

Printed in the United States of America
10 9 8 7 6 5 4 3 2 1

Library of Congress Cataloging-in-Publication Data is available upon request.
ISBN 9781944648664
eISBN 9781944648671

Editing by Alexa Stevenson
Copyediting by Scott Calamar
Proofreading by Michael Fedison and
    Lisa Story
Text design and composition by Kit Sweeney

Interior illustrations by Vanessa Fiori
Front cover design by Ty Nowicki
Jacket design by Sarah Avinger
Printed by Lake Book Manufacturing

Distributed to the trade by Two Rivers Distribution, an Ingram brand
www.tworiversdistribution.com

Special discounts for bulk sales (minimum of 25 copies) are available. Please contact Aida Herrera at aida@benbellabooks.com.

For Cooper, Benjamin, and David:
Thank you for always looking at me as if I can do
anything and making me believe it myself.
This book happened because of your unending love and support.
Thank you for helping me make my dreams come true.

CONTENTS

FOREWORD

BY JENNIFER HUDSON

I still remember the day I met Liz for the first time. I was meeting with executives from Weight Watchers, and they brought Liz along to talk to me about what it would be like on the program. I had lost a good amount of weight on my own but had hit a plateau and just couldn't seem to get past it. I don't know what it was, maybe the fact that we were both Chicago girls, but Liz and I clicked right away. Still, when we started working together a couple of weeks after that meeting, I was shocked by how much she totally got me and where I was coming from—I mean, she was this thin, sporty, "professional weight-loss expert"! But she had been there. She knew what it was like to try to lose weight and fail, or to lose some and gain it all back. She even had a one-year-old son: my son was a newborn at the time, and Liz understood the lack of sleep and the amazing new life I was experiencing as a mom, because she was living it, and that meant a lot to me. She gave me support I didn't even know I was missing.

All my past diet attempts made me pretty smart about what to eat, which is part of why it was so frustrating to still not be where I wanted to be. I'll bet a lot of you can relate—I could probably recite calorie counts in my sleep, but there I was. What Liz helped me do was make these tiny tweaks to my plan that made all the difference. She spent a ton of time talking about small, healthy changes I could make that would not throw my life out of whack, things that seemed almost too easy. I won't lie; I thought she was crazy some of the time. Especially at first, when she told me I could eat all of my favorite foods. No way, I thought. This is never going to get the weight off. So I decided I knew better and made stricter rules for myself. This didn't work at all, of course, and Liz knew exactly what I was doing. She sat me down and asked me to give her way a chance. Trusting her was the best decision I ever made for my health. She helped me understand that awareness was where I needed to focus, being aware of my habits and planning ahead to make it easier to make good choices. She lovingly guided me back to pizza—go ahead and have that pizza, Jen, just make a habit of eating a huge salad before you grab a slice. That salad filled me up enough that it kept me to just one or maybe two pieces. One piece of pizza never made anyone gain weight, it's all the pieces that usually come after it! Actually, Liz even taught me to make my own pizza, and that became a family thing. Now "Make Your Own Pizza Night" is one of my favorite family traditions.

Involving my family was an incredible gift that Liz gave me. She was a great source of support, but she knew I would need more than just her if my weight loss was going to be a lasting thing. The more people around me on my team and in my family who knew what I was doing, and could support me, the better. She started my *entire* extended family across the country losing weight, and I mean I have a *big* family. Together nearly seventy-five of us lost over 2,000 pounds. This incredible system of support made it so that each time I returned home or went to a family gathering, everyone was on the same page. Liz has a great chapter in this book about support, and advice on how to find support or even build your own Target 100 group. Know that it works! With my family all trying to make changes together, it was a lot easier and more fun; our big family meals were suddenly a lot healthier because we were all trying to help each other reach our goals.

My relationship with Liz continues to be one of the most important to my own goal of living a full and healthy life. We connected from that first day in Chicago, and that bond has only grown stronger, even when we're 3,000 miles away from each other. I hope you will let what Liz has to say touch you, that you will really take it in. Rethink this journey, not as another "diet" but a step-by-step life change that will transform so much more than just your weight. Her lessons come from a place of deep understanding, and she cares more than you will ever know. She cheered me on the entire way with loving kindness, and helped me understand that getting weight off wasn't about being perfect, but instead about creating a program—a life—that I could live with. I'm very lucky, and I love what I do, but my life has some challenges. I might have to fly across the globe at the drop of a hat, managing time changes, jet lag, and not knowing where or how to get a healthy meal in a new town or country. I'm always in front of people, and everyone notices my weight. There are long hours and lots of late nights, and I'm always trying to find that balance between taking care of myself, my career, my family. It's not always easy, and I know it won't always be easy for you. But I also know that you can do this!

I am so excited that you have picked up this book. Trust me, Liz has been where you are. To this day I call on her as my dear friend and wise teacher when I need help maintaining my weight and wellness, and Liz always has a solution, and she is always there. She will be there for you, too.

INTRODUCTION
MY STORY

S truggling with weight has been part of my identity for most of my life. I was an overweight child, and I was teased mercilessly. The world is still unkind to women and girls who don't fit the mold, but these days the idea that we should accept different body types is at least gaining traction. Believe me, no one had heard the term "body shaming" in my elementary school in 1983.

I first started trying to lose weight at the age of fourteen, when I was the only kid attending meetings at the local diet center. I lost the weight . . . and then I gained most of it back. Throughout my teens, twenties, and early thirties, I would lose and gain the same thirty-five pounds over and over and over again. I tried every plan imaginable and read every diet book I could get my hands on. I got really good at losing weight, but the number on the scale always, always crept back up.

Unfortunately for me, that number was crucially important to my professional life. As a Broadway actress and singer, I knew that extra pounds could make the difference between landing or losing a part. My body was constantly under intense, open scrutiny. Agents and casting directors thought nothing of telling me I was too heavy for a role—or praising me when I starved myself into a more acceptable state of thinness. I tried just about every crazy deprivation diet, and whatever weight I couldn't starve off I exercised away with extreme workout regimens. Nothing was too radical for me to try. When I noticed how thin most long-distance runners are, I immediately began training for a marathon. My finish time was respectable, but because of my poor eating habits, I became one of the unlucky few who manage to gain weight while training for a marathon!

A story from my late twenties provides a dramatic example of the unhealthy relationship I had with my body. At the time, I had just finished a national tour with *Show Boat*. My weight was low because I had been following a fad diet and burning calories like crazy performing a physically challenging role. A casting call went out for the touring production of *Les Misérables*: I auditioned for the role of Cosette's understudy, and I *killed* it. I was absolutely elated, sure that I'd be chosen. So when weeks went by and I heard nothing, I was crushed. I turned to food for comfort, as I so often had in the past, and my famished body began to pile on weight at a rate that was astonishing even for me. Imagine my surprise when I got a call nearly six months after the audition telling me that the part was now mine . . . and I had just a few weeks to get back to my audition weight. In the history of weight loss, I don't think anyone has ever dropped thirty pounds faster.

My weight had come to define me. My inability to keep weight off once I lost it baffled me, because I felt so miserable when my weight was high and so much more relaxed when it was low. Looking back, I realize that this sense of contentment had less to do with the physical changes that come with weight loss than it did with the mental ones. When I lost weight, I felt like I was in control—of my body and my life. When I was overweight, I felt out of control, and the emotional tension that feeling caused left me anxious and unsettled.

A MIND SHIFT

In my early thirties I turned away from acting—I was recently married, and a life of auditions and brutal tour schedules wasn't what I wanted anymore. Suddenly free of the constant pressure to be thin, I completely let go of all healthy habits. At first, I felt like a prisoner who had been released from a jail she didn't even realize she was in. I gained weight quickly, and as the pounds added up, I began to realize that even without a role to worry about, I didn't like carrying the extra weight I'd put on: I felt heavy and lethargic and uncomfortable in my skin. I couldn't honestly say I was "happy at any weight" or "didn't care about how I looked." Realizing this was both a disappointment and a relief. My internal truth was that I wanted to lose weight regardless of the career path I was on—I didn't need to be rail thin anymore, but at the size I'd reached after a few months of freedom, inhaling ice cream on the couch, I just didn't feel like myself. So I returned to my old standbys, trying one fad diet after another, but as I had gotten older, my extra weight had become more stubborn, and I was no longer willing to completely starve myself or exercise for multiple punishing hours to make up for my slowing metabolism. I decided I needed to shake things up and try something completely new.

In all my years of obsessive dieting, despite adopting nearly every weight-loss craze that came along, I'd somehow managed to avoid perhaps the most ubiquitous weight-loss program of all: Weight Watchers. The reason for this was pretty simple—I was all about the dramatic approach, and Weight Watchers seemed too cautious, too plodding. Why count points and lose a pound or two at a time when you could exist on nothing but cabbage soup for a week and drop two sizes? But I'd seen people close to me have success with the program, and my usual strategies weren't working, so why not? To say that my expectations were low is a huge understatement, but I gave it a try.

I'm glad I did—because it changed the course of my life.

Weight Watchers gave me tools I'd never had before, including a realistic eating plan that was flexible enough for me to follow long term and, most importantly, an amazing support system that helped me give voice to the doubts, fears, and insecurities that had dogged me for so many years. Sharing my experiences, hearing the stories of other members, and receiving encouragement and advice started to heal some of the emotional and physical damage I had sustained during my years of yo-yo dieting. I learned to appreciate progress, even when it was hard to measure. I learned to celebrate the choices I made, even when the results weren't dramatic.

I'd had things backward during my early years. I believed that losing weight was the key to feeling good about myself because it was proof that I was in control. Only now did I realize that this control was an illusion: my weight had been controlling me, not the other way around—it determined how I felt, what I ate, how I talked to myself, how I spent my time. Taking control of my choices about how I treated my body and mind, and divorcing them from the number on the scale—ditching the fad diets, exercising in a joyful way, talking to myself with acceptance and love rather than shame and criticism—would not only help me lose weight for good, but more importantly give me a sense of peace that was unshakeable because it came from the inside.

SECRETS OF SUCCESS

I reached my goal weight, and for the first time in my life, I maintained my weight loss. But Weight Watchers gave me more than a new relationship with my body—it gave me a new career as well. When a receptionist job opened up at a local center, I applied, thinking of it as a temporary thing. I'd spend the next eleven years working at Weight Watchers. I became a meeting leader, and before I knew it, I was running seventeen group-support meetings a week, helping to create the fledgling Weight Watchers website, and interviewing members for articles and videos. Eventually, I went on to become the company's director of brand advocacy.

One of my favorite early jobs at the company was collecting the stories of successful members across the country. To do this, I read tons of letters and email messages from amazing people who'd lost weight on the plan, and selected exceptional stories to feature online and in *Weight Watchers* magazine. Then I'd bring those members to New York City, a dozen at a time, for interviews and video shoots to be used for promotional purposes.

That job was such a gift. It allowed me to talk one-on-one with people who had achieved a goal that, in many cases, they'd been struggling toward for their entire lives—and examine exactly what they had done to reach it at last. Interviewing them gave me an incredible opportunity to delve into the details of what worked—and what didn't—for hundreds and hundreds of weight-loss "success stories." I methodically scrutinized their behaviors, habits, choices, and routines like an anthropologist searching for the secrets of a lost society. I learned many, many lessons from these inspirational men and women, but the biggest one of all was this:

THERE IS NO ONE "BEST WAY" FOR EVERYONE TO LOSE WEIGHT—BUT THERE ARE "BEST WAYS" FOR EACH INDIVIDUAL PERSON TO SUCCEED AT WEIGHT LOSS.

Having a fantastic weight-loss program is a starting point, but it's not enough. In my experience, everyone who figures out how to lose weight and keep it off does so by creating their *own* best program based on their individual personality, preferences, and history. People don't succeed by blindly following a one-size-fits-all diet and exercise plan; they triumph when they begin with a great plan and customize it until it fits them like a glove. Those I interviewed had succeeded not because they slavishly followed the Weight Watchers program point by point, but because they figured out how to adapt it to their own lives.

Once I realized this, I looked back at my own weight-loss history and realized I had spent years following other people's plans without ever making them my own. Every time I lost weight via someone else's cookie-cutter instructions, I'd gain it all back as soon as I started being Liz again. It was by listening to other members at Weight Watchers meetings that I began to see that the only way to lose weight and keep it off for good was to figure out what worked for *me*. Everyone seemed to have their own tricks and methods based on their unique likes and dislikes, their schedules and families. I found myself coming up with my own "hacks," adopting what worked and ditching what didn't, and without really realizing it, I made the program my own.

STAR TREATMENT

Around the time I was making all these breakthroughs, I met David Kirchhoff, then the president and CEO of WeightWatchers.com. David joined the Weight Watchers meeting that I had been asked to run for the dot com side of the business, and we really hit it off. I coached him through a forty-pound weight loss, and that experience solidified a bond that would last through our next ten years working together and beyond.

As celebrities started becoming interested in Weight Watchers, David—his own weight-loss success fresh in his mind—recommended that the company send me out to meet with VIP clients personally. Attending weekly meetings with a trained leader was an integral part of the program, but it wasn't practical for celebrities to pop in at a local center. The thinking was that I would bring the meetings to them and provide one-on-one coaching.

This proved to be a winning strategy: With my help as their personal weight-loss coach, high-profile members had far more success than they did simply trying to follow the program on their own. Eventually, Weight Watchers began referring to me as the company's "secret weapon"—the "fixer" who helped celebrity clients meet their goals. I flew from New York to Los Angeles every week to lead meetings for Jessica Simpson and a dozen of her friends and relatives. I helped Katie Couric figure out how to negotiate the on-set buffet table as a newly minted news anchor. During a late-night phone call, I helped Jennifer Hudson understand that she could indeed fit Buffalo wings into her meal plan. When a VIP client was having trouble with the program, I'd step in and offer guidance and support tailored to their needs.

Personal coaching was giving me a training ground to begin distilling some of my insights about weight loss. I'd started to learn about the science of habit formation, and realized that many of the strategies I'd found most successful relied upon identifying and understanding habits. Meanwhile, I began serving as a media spokesperson for Weight Watchers, appearing on television, sometimes with one of my clients—like Jennifer Hudson, who by then had become a spokesperson herself.

FACE OF THE BRAND

When Jennifer Hudson first joined Weight Watchers, she wasn't aiming to become the brand's spokesperson—she just wanted to lose weight. She had the title role in the upcoming film *Winnie Mandela*, and the producers had asked her to slim down for the part. I was assigned to help her learn the plan, and as fellow Chicago girls and new moms, we bonded right away. But things didn't go perfectly right out of the gate. At first, she didn't lose any weight—in fact, she was gaining. I flew down to see her in Tampa and could tell that the problem was a familiar one: she wasn't convinced that what I was suggesting would work. She assumed dieting had to be difficult, and had some very punishing beliefs about the choices she would have to make in order to lose weight. Just as I had in my younger years, Jennifer believed that to succeed she had to be starving, depriving herself of all the foods she enjoyed, living on nothing but plain chicken breasts and salad. Instead of trusting the program, she was overdoing it, imposing severe restrictions that inevitably backfired after just a few days, when her hunger won out—and then she'd start all over again. I told Jennifer that limiting herself to "diet food" would not get her where she wanted to go. She needed to customize her eating plan—and include foods she actually enjoyed eating—to achieve long-term success.

Jennifer agreed to give my approach a try. "Give me a week," I told her. We stayed in constant contact over those seven days in order to identify and challenge old thought patterns when they arose. I had her eating things she thought would—or should—be off-limits, like sushi and chicken wings. She finally began losing weight: For Jennifer, the magic formula was staying away from severe restrictions that triggered her old feelings about dieting, and instead learning how to incorporate small treats into her everyday life. She could eat well all day if she knew she had chocolate to look forward to in the afternoon.

Jennifer worked so hard. While she was losing the weight, she was busy prepping for her movie role and not in the public eye as much as she had been. Because of this, I think it appeared to many that her weight loss was dramatically fast. This is the magic of marketing. In fact, Jennifer's weight loss was very healthy and very real, and with all the ups and downs that are characteristic of real weight loss. Some weeks she would do everything "right" and still not lose a pound. This is incredibly normal, but also incredibly discouraging. She persevered through those tough days and learned that consistency and determination really do pay off. When she stepped back into the spotlight, it created a frenzy. People were simply astounded at her transformation. Jennifer was and continues to be an inspiration for many struggling to lose weight and keep it off, but she didn't do it just by working within a plan; she did it by making a plan work for her.

UNIVERSAL STRUGGLES, INDIVIDUAL SOLUTIONS

A similar pattern emerged with other celebrities I coached. Following a weight-loss plan wasn't enough to guarantee success: they needed an approach to that plan that was tailored to them as individuals, taking into account their strengths and weaknesses, one that identified and adjusted the behaviors and beliefs that were holding them back.

For example, Jessica Simpson's approach to weight loss was less emotionally guided than Jennifer's—she was all about rational diligence. A typical oldest child, she reminded me of the kid who sits in the front row of class and raises her hand to answer every question. Jessica listened to everything I said, tried every one of my suggestions, and measured and tracked everything she ate. We worked together three times—before her first pregnancy, between her pregnancies, and after her second child was born. Each time, Jessica worked with a methodical focus I've rarely seen in any client, famous or not.

Charles Barkley was totally different. We tried several strategies that didn't work—they didn't fit his personality or his schedule. What he needed was something very simple that didn't involve a lot of time, effort, or thought. Eventually we hit on the perfect fit—we called it his "game plan." We created a list of five breakfasts, five lunches, five dinners, and a handful of snacks that worked well for him—then, for each meal, he simply chose one from the list. For Charles, food was just fuel; he didn't mind the repetition of having only five predetermined options. What mattered to him was not having to think about what he was going to eat—he didn't want to be measuring, adding, or tracking, and his "game plan" was the solution. This approach made sense to his athlete's mind-set, and it fit well into his hectic travel and training schedule.

For Katie Couric, the focus was on fine-tuning. Not only does the path to successful weight loss vary from person to person, it varies over time, and may need to be readjusted as our bodies and circumstances change. As she entered her forties, Katie had begun shifting away from intense exercise and more toward restorative, flexibility-centered activities like yoga and Pilates. I'm a huge fan of both—but they weren't providing the intensive workouts that Katie's body needed to stay slim, build muscle, and amp up her metabolism as she embarked on middle age. So Katie and I set out to revamp her fitness program: We knew she needed a quick, high-intensity workout that fit into her schedule, so she tried all kinds of exercise classes that met those criteria. She fell in love with spinning, and made that the center of her routine. We also tweaked her diet—we need fewer calories as we get older, and unfortunately, even with plenty of exercise, her food choices had to reflect that reality to prevent her from gaining weight.

Before I began working with them, I'd assumed (like most people, probably) that losing weight was easy for celebrities. After all, they had the resources to hire chefs, nutritionists, and trainers. In truth, celebrities face the same basic challenge as everyone else, and it is a big one: Figuring out how to create a diet and exercise plan that they can follow—joyfully—*every day*. Most have some additional challenges I hadn't thought of, like supercharged versions of the universal struggles we all face. My celebrity clients often had crazy, unhealthy schedules and sleep patterns. They were surrounded not only by tempting food, but by people paid to say yes to them. Their weight and appearance were topics of public discussion, and (especially for women) often tied to their career success, producing extreme, counterproductive anxiety.

Working with celebrities further convinced me of the importance of looking closely not just at clients' diet and exercise habits but at their lives as a whole, to find the emotional, behavioral, and environmental barriers standing between them and their goals. Only then could I help them determine what "fixes" might work for them.

When it comes to weight loss, our struggles are universal—but our solutions are individual.

THE NEXT STEP

I left Weight Watchers in 2013. The company had changed, and I'd disagreed with several choices that I felt did not square up with the latest research into processed foods and the optimal intake of carbohydrates, fat, and protein. I had spent over a decade watching the company change lives—including mine—and I will always be a fan, but more personally, I was seeing that I had become a Weight Watchers expert, when what I *really* wanted to be was a weight-loss expert. It was time to move on and push myself to learn new things. I went back to school and became certified as both a personal trainer and a nutrition exercise specialist.

Since then, I've continued to work with all kinds of clients, from celebrities and CEOs to stay-at-home parents, helping them succeed not by introducing radical changes, but by simplifying and customizing their weight-loss strategies, relying on what I've learned about habit formation. I also began consulting across the country in every sector of the weight-loss industry that would have me. My first consulting gig was with Life Time Fitness, helping them create one of their first corporate weight-loss programs, and soon I was consulting for wearable device companies, helping them consider how to incorporate behavior modification techniques into their products. As wellness technology exploded, my work expanded into mobile wellness platforms and incredible new products that would have seemed like science fiction when I first started trying to lose weight as a teenager.

All of this new information, along with my years of experience, has given me a unique perspective on weight loss. I had seen time and time again that the people who achieved permanent weight loss were those who mastered their habits and developed their own plans—but I was also aware that, while some of us intuitively know how to do this, most of us do not. That's where I came in—and where Target 100 comes in. I was ready to develop a program of my own.

At Weight Watchers I'd worked with the scientists, dietitians, and exercise experts who revised and updated the program, leading focus groups to find out what people really wanted and needed from a weight-loss program, and then working to incorporate the science of bodies and behavior into plans and strategies that would make sense to and work for real people. Over and over I heard that people want simplicity in their program, but they also want it to be flexible, and a little bit fun. The comments from those focus groups rang in my ears as I set out to create my own plan, as did the lessons I'd learned from culling success stories, from coaching individual clients, from studying habit science and building new programs and new technologies. I put every bit of my experience into the development of Target 100.

My clients trust me, in part because they know that I don't just talk the talk, I walk the walk with them every day. I faced fifty-pound and sixty-five-pound weight-loss hurdles, respectively, after the births of my sons. I struggle through highs and lows as I continue to maintain my weight loss, and because of this I understand my clients in a way many others do not. My personal weight-loss strategies have changed over the years, and I continue

Put *you* into your weight-loss program. Don't let anyone else dictate how you will change your own life.

to fine-tune them, applying new knowledge to my own life just as I put it into action with my clients. The plan I follow has evolved as I've gotten older, had children, changed my exercise goals, and so on. This evolution is the soul of Target 100: continuing to personalize our own weight-loss plans is the key to continuing success.

Over the course of this book, I will guide you in creating a foolproof weight-loss plan that fits your personality, schedule, health goals, and lifestyle. Within these pages you'll find the specific, personal advice you need to solve the mystery of weight loss and address the issues that have held you back in the past. The book is filled with clear explanations and concrete strategies, plus exercises and worksheets that you will never regret filling out. I have journaled through nearly every weight-loss attempt I have made over the years—the successful and the frustrating—and I am glad that I did. I look back on these journals for reminders of what's worked (and what hasn't!) and to access motivation when it is running low. Take the time to write notes in the margins of this book—highlight passages, bookmark pages, make it your own.

When we set out to lose weight following a standardized program— whatever it is—we tend to assume that if the program doesn't work, it's because we have failed. I wholeheartedly disagree with this. If a weight-loss plan doesn't work, it's the plan that needs fixing, not the person. My goal—in life and in this book—is to help you create your own success: to identify which tools work best, which habits need unlearning, which thinking processes need reframing. I won't tell you what to eat; I'll give you the information you need to experiment and discover what works best for you. I will inspire, inform, and motivate, but while I am the author of this book, ultimately you will be the author of your plan. If you've tried to lose weight before, I'll bet you've invested a lot of time in memorizing rules and food lists, point values and calories. Target 100 asks you to try something different. Allow yourself to put more time into understanding yourself than into understanding a program designed by someone else.

Losing weight should be about self-discovery, not blind devotion to somebody else's rules. Once I truly understood this, I felt driven to share what I had learned. Target 100 is the result.

GETTING STARTED

THE BASICS

Chapter 1

HABIT AND ENVIRONMENT—YOUR

SECRET WEAPON IS YOURSELF

W hen I start working with private clients, I tell them the first session will be an hour and a half instead of the usual hour. They understand this initial meeting is vital because it is when I will explain the foundations of the program, and walk them through the tools they will need to master in order to succeed. But that foundation, and these tools, are never what they are expecting. They show up expecting to hear about a food plan and exercise regime—basically assuming that I will tell them what to do and what to eat to lose the weight. Instead, I begin by explaining why that approach hasn't worked in the past, and why it won't work now. This chapter is my nod to that first client meeting. I want you to let go of your ideas about what a diet book should be and come at this with a fresh set of eyes and an open mind.

What if I told you that you are basically not present for over half of the health decisions you make in a day? That they are not really decisions at all? In fact, they are habits—habits so ingrained that you likely don't even know you have them. Uncovering these and triggering new, more conscious involvement in your choices is what will remove the barriers that have kept you from success. Target 100 is built on a set of holistic guidelines in six areas (nutrition, hydration, exercise, movement, stress, and sleep). These guidelines can be life changing. But without the engine of habit change behind them, they are just another set of rules that can't (and won't) be followed long term. Let me be very clear: **Understanding and applying the formula for changing habits is the only way to achieve lasting weight loss.** This is where—and why—most plans fail. There is lots of telling you what to do and very little explaining how to do it. The reassurance I find myself giving to clients—so often that it has become my catchphrase—is: *You are not broken*. People come to me bewildered and in despair, asking:

"Why is it that I can accomplish so many other things in my life, but this one goal defeats me again and again?" It's not because they are "weak," it's because they've been using the wrong tools—imagine if you tried to pound a nail into the wall using a screwdriver! They've been using the wrong tools because for years they've been urged to fight the wrong enemy: the fight is not with *food*, it is with *habits*.

In this chapter, we will learn the formula for habit change, and in every chapter after this, we will apply it. It is the glue that will make this plan stick. The best part? You can use this simple formula to change more than just your weight or even your health—you can use it to change any behavior that isn't getting you what you want.

UNDERSTANDING HABITS

Habits affect more than just your health decisions: it has been estimated that up to 45 percent of everything we do in the course of a given day is habitual. So, what is a habit? As defined in *Webster's Dictionary*, a habit is "an acquired mode of behavior that has become nearly or completely involuntary." Have you ever driven a car only to arrive at your destination with no recollection of the drive itself? That is what is meant by "involuntary behavior." As hard as it is to believe, nearly half of what you do every single day is rote behavior that you repeat on a kind of autopilot, triggered by an assortment of emotional and sensory cues.

Take your morning routine. If you were to actually pay attention to the way you brush your teeth, you would notice that you do it almost *exactly* the same way each time. From the way you hold the toothbrush, to which side of your mouth you start on, to how you stand and spit and rinse, it is all perfectly choreographed. When you hop in the shower, you probably have a similarly predictable routine for how you wash and dry yourself. Most of the time I am totally unaware of what I am doing in the shower: my mind is elsewhere, on the day ahead or lost in other thoughts. My body mindlessly carries me through the motions. An interesting exercise is to take note of your own shower routine and then try to change one piece of it. For instance, I noticed that when I shower, I always shave my right leg before my left. Every time. When I decided to begin shaving my left leg first as an experiment, it was amazing how difficult it was. First off, I kept forgetting! I'd remember after I was already halfway done shaving my right leg. Then, on the days when I did remember, it just felt *weird*. There is really nothing more logical about starting with the right leg than with the left, but not to felt wrong somehow. I didn't like it; I wanted to go back to the "old way" I was comfortable with. And yet shaving is very different from habits involving food. There aren't biological, hormonal urges driving me, and there is certainly no guilt or shame wrapped up in the way I shower. Think about how much more difficult it might be to change habits entangled with those additional factors.

Your brain works hard to create habits so that you do not have to make the same decisions over and over again. For instance, what if you had to decide how to shave and how to brush your teeth each and every morning? You'd be wasting important decision-making energy you need for the more complex parts of your day, and so your brain tries to conserve that energy by relegating decisions like this to the realm of habit. This isn't just a metaphor: Our logical thinking takes place in the frontal cortex—your brain keeps that vital space from being tied up by shunting habitual actions to an entirely different part of the brain. This is a good thing! It is why you can think and perform other tasks at the same time.

Your habits are imprinted on your brain as neural shortcuts, and the more you habitually do something the stronger that pathway becomes. Think of it like a road: As you perform a habit over and over, the road gets smoother and wider, easier and more automatic to travel. This is why trying to simply "do things differently" via brute force is so seldom successful. To create a new, fledgling habit, it must be burned into a neural pathway; at first it will feel like driving over a rough dirt road, and your brain would always rather default to the well-worn path.

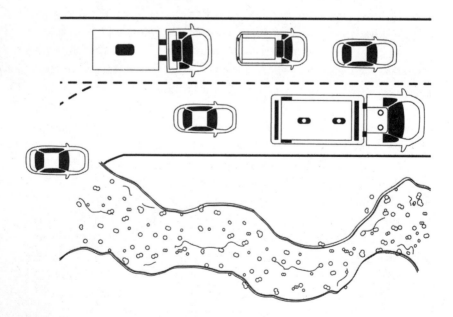

And yet we believe we can alter behaviors that have been with us for years by simply following a new meal plan! Changing your habits is a skill, one that requires you not only to learn to recognize them, but also to understand how they work.

THE HOW OF HABITS

Let's look at the anatomy of a habit. Habits are set in motion by what's called a "trigger" or a cue. That trigger can be anything from a time of day (morning = brush my teeth) to a physical sensation (yucky morning taste in my mouth = brush my teeth) to an emotional response (tired and trying to wake myself up = brush my teeth) to a simple thought pattern (just had coffee, should brush my teeth). Triggers are all around us, in our environment and our near-unconscious thoughts, but they go mostly unnoticed. The trigger prompts a behavior, and over time, if the pair is repeated, the trigger comes to be strongly connected to the behavior, which becomes a habit. To use one of the examples above, you might be triggered to brush your teeth after having coffee by thinking you should. But unless you keep repeating the practice of brushing your teeth after you have coffee, it will not become a habit.

Once a habit is triggered, we move into the "routine" part of a habit's anatomy—for instance, the actual action of brushing our teeth. This then leads to the habit's final piece, which is the "reward" we get from the routine. When we brush our teeth, that reward is a clean feeling, better breath, and so on.

Taken together, these three pieces make up what we will call "the habit loop."

When we think of a habit, the second piece of its anatomy, the routine, is generally what we think of, but in fact, the other two pieces drive our actions. By the time it is habit, the routine is mostly involuntary. It is only by recognizing the other parts of its anatomy—the triggers in particular—that we can step in and change a habit.

Now, brushing our teeth is a good habit—but not all of our habits are good. And habits can be nested together with other habits and become hard to untangle. Perhaps you have a bad habit of waking up too late to eat a healthy breakfast, which leaves you rushing to work, where there is a donut shop in the basement. That lateness habit is a trigger itself. The stress, lack of preparation, and lack of time kick off a routine of stopping at the donut shop, one you continually fall prey to once it is established because it also comes with a powerful reward. That sugary donut is delicious: it gives you a quick burst of energy in the morning, and it gets happy chemicals flowing after the stress of being late, providing what feels like a much-needed treat

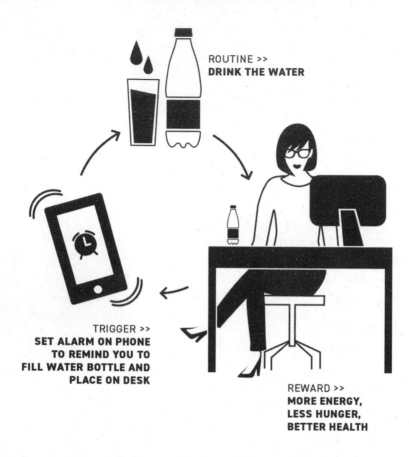

ROUTINE >>
DRINK THE WATER

TRIGGER >>
**SET ALARM ON PHONE
TO REMIND YOU TO
FILL WATER BOTTLE AND
PLACE ON DESK**

REWARD >>
**MORE ENERGY,
LESS HUNGER,
BETTER HEALTH**

before the long workday begins. Traditional diets would tell you: "Hey, just start eating eggs for breakfast." Unfortunately, this doesn't address the root of the problem (your trouble waking up on time) or the fact that eating eggs for breakfast instead of running out the door requires myriad new tasks and behaviors including shopping for eggs or other ingredients, getting up early enough to make breakfast, and finding a way to make this new routine feel rewarding so that you stick with it long enough for it to become a habit. Knowing you should eat a healthier breakfast doesn't get you very far—you might succeed in keeping at it for a short time, but once the novelty fades or you hit a bump in the road, you'll revert to your old habit, because the new routine wasn't properly planned for and supported.

The good news is that you are not beholden to your habits. *Any* habit can be untangled and broken with the right combination of awareness and skill—and there is really nothing you can't make into a habit if you want to.

Habit formation is the process by which a behavior, through regular repetition, becomes automatic or routine. The magic is in the repetition and in consistency. Consistency is not the same thing as perfection—interestingly, perfection is much less important. In a recent study of habit formation, missing a day of performing the behavior mattered less than whether participants returned to performing it the very next day. In short, what will matter as you are building new, healthier habits for weight loss isn't whether you "slip up," it's what you do afterward—whether you pick yourself up and keep trying.

The habit of perfectionism is a success killer. My advice? Go ahead, give yourself permission to be mediocre! It works—and it's a lot more fun!

The same study also revealed that the average time it took for a behavior to become automatic was 66 days—with a range of 18 to 254 days. This speaks volumes: there is no one-size-fits-all-habits timeline. Some habits will be relatively easy to break or build, while others will be harder, have more layers, and take more time. Rome wasn't built in a day—and neither are habits. Target 100 doesn't promise a "21 Days to Flat Abs" type of solution. What I can promise, though, is that the success you achieve this way will *actually last*. I am also 100 percent confident in *you*. Whatever your past failures or personal challenges, I promise you are not somehow the one person out of the thousands I've worked with who just "can't." You've got this.

Breaking old habits and creating new ones are two sides of the same coin, and an especially effective way to tackle either is to replace a habit that already exists with something different. Maybe your problem is oversleeping and grabbing that breakfast donut, or maybe it is late-night eating—for my friend Katie, it was a long-standing habit of eating dessert every day after lunch. Katie's habit was one that she'd developed as a child: In her home, they always ate dessert after lunch. Even when she took a packed lunch to school, it always included a dessert. Katie knew this practice was standing in the way of her weight-loss progress, but it was tied up in emotional and habitual knots.

To tackle this habit, we first identified its parts. Katie's trigger was lunch. Each day she ate lunch and each day, immediately afterward, she had dessert. Even the time of day had become a trigger—she found herself thinking of dessert as soon as she noticed midday approaching. The routine, of course, was the actual behavior of eating dessert right after lunch. The reward was

> **Identifying Triggers.** A habit's trigger is anything that's encouraging it, or making it "go." Habits can have multiple triggers! Some things to consider:
>
> - Environment and location—Are there outside cues for the habit, like a sight or smell, or being in a certain place?
> - Stressors or emotions—Are there emotions that seem to lead to the behavior?
> - Physical state—Are you hungry or tired when you perform this habit?
> - Time of day—Is the habit tied to a particular time or event?
> - Relationship associations—Is this habit cued by a relationship that repeats certain patterns? Does your husband's habit of eating ice cream to cope with work stress lead you to join him? Do you always meet a particular friend at a bar?

the sweet treat itself, and perhaps having something to look forward to, a moment of indulgence in the middle of the day to escape stress. Now, as we saw in the earlier examples of swapping donuts for eggs at breakfast or switching up my leg-shaving routine, just telling herself to stop eating dessert after lunch won't cut it for Katie, not long term. Instead, she must use the habit loop to trigger a new routine that will get her the same reward, or another one that is just as desirable. So, knowing Katie would otherwise forget, we set a timer on her phone for around lunchtime that reminded her *not* to have a treat after lunch. The new routine was eating lunch without dessert. The reward we came up with was that for each day Katie avoided the old habit, she could put two dollars in a jar for new clothes. This gave her the same feeling of "treating herself" that she got from dessert.

It may take some trial and error to find a reward that works for you. For some habits, and some people, the natural rewards—feeling better, having more energy, losing weight—are immediate or compelling enough that no extra thought is needed. Or the routine itself is so effortless and divorced from emotion that all you really need is a trigger. Other times, especially if you are at a place in your process where results are slow, you will need to experiment to find a healthier replacement for an old routine that still provides the reward you are looking for. You may find the reward you decide to use doesn't quite hit the spot—sometimes you *think* you know what you are getting from a habit, but in reality the reward is something else. In cases like this, you may have to go back and try a new reward until you hit on something that fits. Maybe replacing your afternoon croissant with a less carb-heavy serving of dark chocolate didn't work, because while you thought the reward of the croissant was the indulgent sweet, it was actually getting up from your desk and walking to the bakery, getting a break from work.

Another important point is that many habits have tasks associated with them that you will need to complete before they can be set in motion—for instance, if your goal is to begin eating healthy dinners at home instead of grabbing takeout on the way home from work, you will need to ensure that you have healthy food in the house.

Below is a template you can use to work out the details of any habit change you decide to make.

THE HABIT CHANGE KEY

Identify the habit you want to change:

_____

Figure out the trigger that is setting that habit in motion:

_____

Identify the reward you are getting from that habit:

_____

Create a new trigger:

_____

Insert a new routine:

_____

Identify whether your routine is supplying the same or an equally desirable reward, and what that reward is:

_____

List the tasks you will need to complete before you kick off this new habit:

_____

_____

_____

TAKING EMOTION OUT OF THE PROCESS

There are two ways emotion affects the weight-loss process. One is that emotion can drive habits and food choices. Often we have a set of habits built around our emotions so that feeling the emotion prompts an immediate desire to eat or to do something to either escape that emotion or augment it—to soothe or celebrate. It's as automatic as following "shave and a haircut" with "two bits." For example, if you head to the vending machines every time your stress levels rise at work, pretty soon it becomes an ingrained habit. Stress hits, and you are standing with your mouth watering and your hand reaching to pull the candy from the machine before you really know what you're doing. Does this sound like you?

For me, it wasn't a vending machine, it was a glass of wine. I worked all day while my husband, a Broadway actor, worked all night. I would arrive home from work, exhausted, to manage dinner and homework and bedtime for two kids all on my own. There was not one second of transition time—I was off to the races. Stressed and lonely, I started pouring myself a glass of wine every night around 6 PM. It relaxed me a little and made me less irritable. Unfortunately, it also made me more likely to snack while making dinner, and eventually I began to suspect it was interfering with my weight maintenance. That was a tough habit to break. It was being triggered both by emotion and by time of day—once the habit was solidified, just seeing the sun set in the sky could turn my thoughts to that glass of wine. As I set out to break the habit, I realized another problem was that we stored opened bottles in plain sight, white in the fridge where it was the first thing you saw on opening the door, and red right out on the kitchen counter. Just seeing the bottle was a trigger (and not needing to pull out the corkscrew made it that much easier to pour myself a glass). So my first move was to move the bottles! Then I set an alarm on my phone with a reminder to go upstairs each night around 6 PM. I needed to busy myself in an area that did not trigger the habit while performing a task that would give me the same feeling I was getting from the wine. The wine was calming, and sipping it made me feel like I was carving out a little space just for myself. Cleaning and organizing gave me a similar feeling, and getting upstairs—alone, where it was quieter—took my stress level down. I realized that however busy I was, I could afford fifteen minutes to decompress, and so every night when the alarm sounded I went upstairs and did something soothing and orderly, like folding laundry—sometimes I called my sister for a chat at the same time. Just that brief distraction was enough to break the habitual loop that had been running and set a new one in motion. (Incidentally, this is another example that shows why it's so important to personalize your plan and your approach to habits and rewards—not everyone, I am aware, finds folding laundry relaxing! Yet knitting, which is calming for some people I know, would probably have sent me stomping back to the wine bottle in frustration.)

Let me be real with you: breaking a habit can feel terrible. I alluded to this a bit when I talked about my shaving experiment. However, especially for habits with emotion attached to them, it can be more than just uncomfortable—it can kick up some powerful emotional resistance. At first, even though I knew I wanted to

Shifting the focus from food to habits and their triggers debunks the idea that lack of success is due to some intrinsic flaw or a deficiency of willpower. And that changes everything.

change my 6 PM wine habit, I felt like a petulant child when the alarm went off. It felt unfair that I couldn't have everything I wanted (weight loss with unlimited wine intake!), and I struggled to stay upstairs and focus on my new routine. Expect a flood of emotions that make you think you *need* the old habit. You will probably be crabby! I know I certainly was—but then one night I realized that I wasn't even thinking about the wine anymore. I had arrived! And believe me, the surge of satisfaction when you conquer a habit is amazing. You will feel unstoppable—confident and excited about your abilities.

So, emotionally driven habits are one way emotion affects the weight-loss process. The second way is through the feelings we have about ourselves. Most damaging, from my perspective, is how we feel about our perceived failures in past attempts to lose weight. For some reason, the only person we ever blame for failure in this area is ourself. Even when clients have joined expensive weight-loss programs and paid for help losing weight, most never blame the program if it doesn't work out. I get it; this was me for many years. We see our weight totally as a matter of personal responsibility—and personal shame. Best of all, we get to wear this "failure" where everyone can see it. Unfortunately, research has emerged to show that the emotions of guilt and shame literally work against us. They activate the reward center in the brain, releasing a burst of the same feel-good chemicals as food, drugs, and sex. Crazy, right? You can see how we might get into a cycle of this behavior, like a rat pushing a lever for a treat. Making a "bad" food choice not only gets us the reward of the food—when we guilt ourselves about that choice, we "rev up" the reward center further, and then we are driven to repeat this again and again.

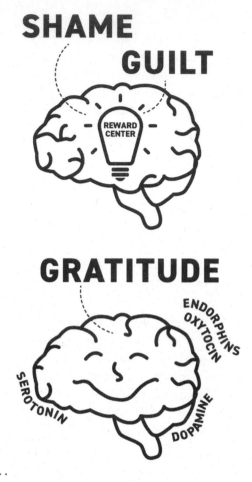

For example: Amy goes to a party where she promises herself she won't drink. She caves to some social pressure and has two glasses of wine. The next day she awakens to feelings of guilt and shame and finds herself craving pancakes . . . almost without thinking she's on her way to the diner for another "hit" of reward chemicals. She has unknowingly been triggered by guilt to seek out her favorite habitual reward: "shameful" food!

I have done this so many times. I would make a mistake and then reward myself with another one. So how can we change something so biological? Well, all habits are biological to some extent—just as with any other habit, we learn to recognize it and use our new knowledge to change it. Another important discovery in the same research was that the act of being grateful—for anything, big or small—actually releases serotonin, dopamine, oxytocin, and endorphins in levels comparable to a low dose of antidepressants. We can change our moods and our minds by creating the simple habit of gratitude. Practicing gratitude can help us neutralize guilt and shame.

If Amy had awakened with a grateful thought (such as: "I am so grateful I only had two glasses instead of four"), she could have jumped back into her healthy routine and been right on track again. Because, to be honest, you can have a couple of "slipups" in a week and still lose weight. But not if you turn each small slipup into an avalanche of bad choices.

Realizing that my brain was wired to respond this way alleviated a lot of guilt about my past mistakes. Suddenly I could release all the negative self-talk that had swirled around this process for so long. When I explain to clients how their habits and environment are colluding to confound them, there is both relief and hope. By beginning to look at weight loss not as a test of character but as a bundle of habits to unravel and master, we also begin to divorce the process from emotion. We can let go of the past, and start from just exactly where we are at this moment.

Letting go of the past doesn't mean erasing it. After all, those past attempts at losing weight were not for nothing: I'll bet you learned and carry forward at least one thing from every attempt you've made. Perhaps you picked up a breakfast smoothie recipe that you use to this day; maybe you found out you love cauliflower while doing a soup diet. At the very least, you've gathered valuable information about what *doesn't* work for you, and what your specific challenges are. All of those past attempts have laid the groundwork for where you are today, and the knowledge you gained will become a piece of your new, personalized, *successful* program.

CREATING HABITS WITH CHARLES BARKLEY

As I started working with Charles Barkley, it became obvious that he was hampered by a bunch of habits that he had been able to get away with when his life was more active, but that were beginning to catch up with him now that he was off the court. One of these was skipping breakfast on his early travel days. As a professional basketball player, he had gotten into the habit of going without breakfast so he could get more sleep—getting overly hungry set him up for overeating later in the day, but this wasn't really a problem when he was a kid burning thousands of calories in practice and games. Unfortunately, it definitely did not serve him well now.

In order to trigger Charles to take food along on his travel days, I looked for something he could "tie" the habit to, something that was already occurring every time he traveled. Charles *loves* watches. I discovered that when he packed for a trip, he always laid out two or three watches to bring along. So, we triggered him to pack some almonds, healthy bars, and oatmeal packets in his carry-on every time he packed his watches. We even bagged up little snack sets that lived in his pantry so that he could just grab one to throw in his bag. As time went by, it became automatic to pack his "emergency rations" every time he packed his watches. This got him through his travel day without grabbing fast food or sugary snacks, and he arrived at his destination well fed and able to make smarter choices throughout the day.

TEN TIPS FOR BREAKING AND BUILDING HABITS

Before I move on to talking about environment, I want to leave you with ten of my most helpful pieces of advice for creating lasting habit change. Take these in, and refer back to them when you get stuck on a particular habit.

1. **Create barriers.** Barriers create awareness. For many clients, it is helpful to build some sort of barrier between them and the habit they want to break. If you are prone to nighttime snacking on the living-room couch, go upstairs at night so that you'd have to walk down to the kitchen to get something to eat. Sometimes, even closing the door or turning out the light in the kitchen at a certain point every evening can be enough— having to open the door or flip that switch gives your brain just enough time to remind you that you're trying to break the habit. If you want to break yourself of the habit of binge-watching television shows, turn off "autoplay" on your streaming service and move the remote across the room. If you want to stop after one serving of dinner, put the leftovers in the fridge before you sit down to eat. Anything that makes the old habit even a tiny bit more difficult can save you from yourself.

2. **Out of sight, out of mind.** Hide everything that is at all tempting to you. There are almost certainly tempting things in your home, especially if you have to live with other humans, as many of us do. Take the time to empty a cupboard (preferably one that is hard to reach—see the previous tip about barriers) and use it to store all things tempting. If you don't have to see it, you will have much better success avoiding it.

3. **Distraction is key.** If you feel yourself pulled toward the thing you are trying to avoid, find a distraction to take your mind off it. Pick up the phone and call a friend, step outside for a brief walk, or get started on a task that needs completing. It's hard to snack mindlessly when you're washing dishes or taking the dog for a run.

4. **Attach one habit to another.** Make building new habits easier by attaching them to actions or habits that are already in place (as Charles Barkley did by packing snacks with his watches). If you are trying to remember to take your vitamins daily, attach this to the act of brushing your teeth. Place the vitamins next to where you keep your toothbrush and begin taking them every day as soon as you finish brushing. It requires less effort to extend an already existing habit than to create a new one from scratch.

5. **Lower the bar.** Habit scientist BJ Fogg has discovered that habits are created when motivation meets action—but action at its smallest, easiest level. Look for ways to break more complex habits, especially those that occur at multiple times of day, into parts, and start with something that requires as little effort as possible. Instead of taking on a habit like "tracking food" all at once, begin by tracking one meal per day until that habit is firmly, reliably established. Having success with an easy first step will create the momentum you need to tackle the next level of your habit change.

6. **Watch the changing seasons.** Each season has built-in triggers and habits associated with it. As the seasons change during your weight-loss process, you may notice forgotten habits rearing their ugly heads. Awareness is key. Keep your eyes peeled for trends and habits unique to a certain season. These might include a tendency to exercise less and drink less water in the winter, eating out more often during a hectic sports-season schedule, or craving foods you associate with a specific time of year. (Pumpkin spice, anyone?)

7. **Remember, habits are smaller than you think.** A habit is a *serial response* to a trigger. Each of those responses can be tiny, and just as it helps to lower the bar by beginning with the *easiest* version of a habit, you will be most successful if you reduce a habit to its smallest part, a small action that will help the larger habit grow. Take something like "drink more water." Lowering the bar might mean beginning by adding just one big tumbler of water to your day. Reducing a habit to its smallest part might look like simply triggering yourself (with an alarm or sticky note) to fill your water tumbler as you arrive at the office each day. That small, concrete change will get you farther than trying to create a habit out of something as vague as "drink more water."

8. **Wait a minute or ten.** When discomfort sets in during a habit change, try setting an alarm for one to ten minutes. Force yourself to sit through the emotional wave of discomfort for those minutes—and watch as the wave passes and you become able to push through the moment. (It really works, I promise!) The more you do this, the more confidence you will gain, and the less time you will need on the clock.

9. **Beware the emotional stages of habit change.** Expect changing a habit to come with emotions—even sitting through a one- to ten-minute waiting period, for instance, you may feel everything from pride to anger to frustration to sadness. If you can become aware of your emotional process, it will become more predictable over time. I have done this

so many times that I know a habit change will result in a predictable (habitual!) progression of thoughts and emotions that always ends with me feeling great about myself for getting through it. Knowing that sense of happiness and pride is waiting for me on the other side has now become a strong motivator for the habit change itself.

10. **Triggers are everything.** No new habit is likely to take hold—or happen at all—if we don't trigger it. Triggers are simply awareness-building moments that remind us of the new routine we would like to make into a habit. Taking a deep look into what is triggering an old habit is what will allow you to break it. Trigger your new habit with something bold and hard to overlook.

THE ENVIRONMENTAL EFFECT

I don't mean to make you paranoid, but I need you to understand that the weight-loss deck is stacked against you. If you don't begin to notice the ways in which your environment is triggering you to eat, you will remain powerless in the face of these influences. Everywhere you turn these days you are confronted with food—food in places it never was before. For example, since when is there food available (chocolate, to be exact) in the swimwear section of department stores? Since some savvy marketer realized that women, stressed by swimsuit shopping, were vulnerable to that impulse

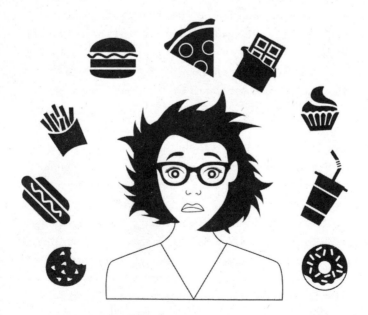

purchase! On top of it all, our genetics are in on it: We are driven to eat by a deep-seated secondary hunger system that compels us to consume food when it is available, even if we are not physically hungry.

If you have ever felt like a marionette on a string, eating for reasons you cannot even explain, examining your internal and external environments will be game changing. I hope you begin to feel like you have been dropped into the Matrix, or like you have a pair of X-ray glasses illuminating all of the insidious traps being set for us day in and day out. The good news? The ability to see these traps is one of the most powerful weight-loss tools there is.

A PHYSICAL RESPONSE

Most people don't realize that, when it comes to food, what we see, smell, feel, and talk about can be just as powerful a drive as true physical hunger. This secondary hunger system—what I call "faux hunger"—was what helped us survive the brutal conditions experienced by our primitive ancestors. If they could overeat when food was plentiful, they could live on their fat stores during inevitable periods of scarcity. The brutal conditions have disappeared, but the system is still with us: you have likely seen it at work when the dessert cart comes around at a restaurant and you go from certain you could not take another bite to hearing yourself order the cheesecake. I named this my "second stomach." Just when I thought I was full, the cookies would be passed around the table and I suddenly had room! Our secondary hunger system can be triggered by any of a number of food cues—images, sounds, and smells.

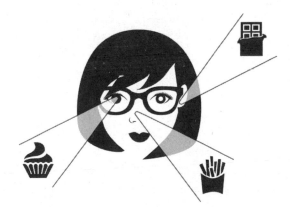

Yup. When we are presented with an image of food, even if we have just eaten, it can spur a seemingly real hunger that manifests with all of the physical signals you get when you are *actually* hungry (like your stomach growling and your mouth watering). This is particularly true for images of high-fat or sugary foods. Fats and sugars prompt a strong response from the brain's pleasure centers; even a billboard that flashes by as you drive can kick off a subliminal feeling of need for them.

TAKING ADVANTAGE OF THE SECONDARY HUNGER SYSTEM

Take a moment to think about all the times you were confronted with a food decision today. You probably think there were just a few, at each of your meals and snacks. Believe it or not, research now proves that you'll most likely make around 200 food decisions today alone. Little did you know that every image, mention, or smell of food set off a complicated decision-making process along with your complex physical reaction to that food cue. How many ads for food did you see today, on television or your computer? How many restaurants did you pass? How many stores did you visit that had tempting goodies at the checkout counter? Yes, every one of those was a food decision. You may not have consciously thought it through, but your brain had to decide whether or not you would pick up that candy bar at checkout. If you didn't, great—but that food cue still gave rise to a secondary hunger signal, one that will help drive your decisions later in the day.

Food itself has changed in recent years—all because food manufacturers want to fatten their bottom line, even if it means fattening millions of us along the way. Food chemists use cutting-edge science to develop addictive new flavors, creating cravings for things we never craved before. Chemical encapsulation of sugar into fat molecules, for example, can make buttery-sweet foods, like cookies, taste better to us than ever. There are foods actually designed to trick us into eating more, beyond fullness and beyond our needs. Companies want us to become conditioned to overeat because once that habit is established, it is a persistent one. Ultimately, food manufacturers have an obligation to stockholders to maximize profits, and the more you eat, the more they sell. There is a word for the food-centric environment that has been evolving steadily since the 1950s. It is called "obesogenic," meaning that the environment itself causes, or contributes to, obesity.

Not too long ago, snacks could only be found in a few places—grocery stores, convenience stores, movie theaters, and so on—making it easier to avoid them. What's more, they were smaller and contained fewer addictive additives. Today, candy, chips, soda, and other low-nutrient, high-carb temptations are sold nearly everywhere, from Old Navy to Home Depot, from Best Buy to the Gap. Nonfood retailers have discovered that they can make big money by placing snacks near checkout counters, with the result that nearly every time we wait in line we are surrounded by food. We're also bombarded with food advertisements, not just on TV, but on our computers and ever-present smartphones. As a result, we must make hundreds of choices every day that didn't exist even a decade ago about whether and what to buy and consume. Scientists now know that as our day goes on and we are called upon to make more and more decisions—not just about food, but about everything—we begin to suffer from "decision fatigue." It is no coincidence that so many of us have such trouble with late-night eating. Over the course of the day it becomes harder and harder to make decisions—and we give in more easily to temptation.

While you have been reading this chapter, learning about habits and the ways in which we can trigger positive behavior change in ourselves, large food and beverage companies have been studying and testing ways of triggering us to eat. They have invested millions in understanding your habits. They tie their products to certain behaviors or times of day, hoping to become part of your daily routine. All of your senses are involved in habit formation, so they use commercials that stimulate your eyes and ears, and even suffuse their shops with certain smells. They target their advertisements for the times and places that research shows you are most likely to succumb. They play on your emotions and even leverage guilt to stoke the brain's reward center. Begin to notice these cues, how you react to them, and what habits they are helping you form.

CHECK YOUR TRIGGERS

When and how are you being triggered? What are your toughest times of the day—when either environmental or emotional stresses make you vulnerable to temptation? List three examples:

_____

_____

_____

I try to look at this as a game. Can I walk into a store and identify all the subtle ways in which I am being triggered to buy or eat? Seeing it as a game makes me more likely to jump in and play to win for myself.

FIGHTING TEMPTATION WITH HABIT

My client Rose has a job she loves that requires an hour-long commute into New York City two or three days a week. As we began to work together, it became obvious that this commute was a weight-loss land mine. From the moment she left her home in the morning, she was challenged by donuts and coffee carts, bagels and stress. In order for Rose to succeed, we first needed to examine every detail of her routine on the days she commuted into the city. Each day on arrival, Rose took the subway and exited up the same set of stairs, where she passed a favorite coffee shop—with amazing pastries. Over time she had created a habit of "treating" herself to one (or two). Sometimes she treated herself because she had a stressful meeting ahead, sometimes to celebrate an accomplishment, other times just because! Rose was aware that the pastries weren't exactly helping her lose weight, but she found herself in the shop making excuses again and again. Rose had created a powerful environment-driven habit.

Traditional weight-loss programs would expect that Rose, now on a diet, should simply stop buying herself pastries, relying on willpower and hope to make it happen. Instead, we went to work making sure she was no longer confronted with the temptation at all. On the next commute day, we set an alarm on her phone for around the time she would arrive at the subway stop. The alarm reminded Rose to head to a different staircase to exit the station. If she never had to pass the shop, she would never have to contend with the physical faux hunger reactions drawing her to the pastries. It would dramatically increase her chances of success. Simply changing her route to avoid seeing the shop or smelling the sweet smell wafting from it was both easier and more effective than white-knuckling her way by it every day. The alarm was crucial to breaking an ingrained transit routine—without that trigger, she would at best have found it more difficult and, more likely, would have forgotten her staircase-change entirely.

BUILDING YOUR MOAT

Think of yourself as a castle that needs a formal layer of protection. In order to fortify you against the bombardments of our obesogenic environment, we will build you a moat of habits and behaviors that will keep you safe. We will build layers of internal and external protections. The larger the moat, the more difficult it will be for the enemy to get across.

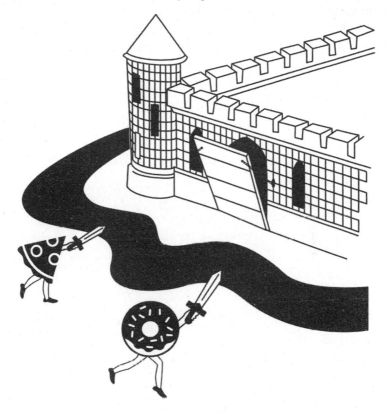

Just as Rose changed her route to work, you will find ways to make the work of changing habits easier. The way you prepare for your day, the way you arrange your environment, and the way you create awareness of your surroundings and your own body will all help determine your success.

Understanding Hunger Signals

The secondary hunger system drove my weight back up again and again until I learned to recognize and differentiate between types of hunger. Recognizing hunger is part of understanding your most important environment—your internal one. It is your first line of defense in the weight-loss battle, and an important part of your moat. I've found that confidence runs low in this area; clients don't trust that they can learn to identify whether they are "really hungry." Getting to know what true hunger and satiety (satisfaction) feel like may take a little practice, but it is absolutely doable and well worth the effort.

I've found that we have three distinct types of hunger. One is true *physical hunger*—this is the one we should feed with actual food. *Not* feeding actual hunger, or letting ourselves get too hungry, can cause just as many problems as eating when we're not really hungry at all. Secondly, we have *emotional hunger*, which drives us to eat food to escape or even amplify an emotion. We can manage this type of hunger by learning to identify which emotion we are feeling and addressing it in another way—for instance, if I am anxious, I may be able to obtain the same stress relief I'm seeking from food by going out for a walk. The third type of hunger is our old friend *faux hunger*. This is pseudo-hunger spurred by the sight, smell, or mention of tempting foods. Let's explore ways to recognize these various hunger types.

- **Physical hunger:** Sets in slowly over time and is satisfied by healthy foods. Any food will do. When you open the fridge, everything looks good. Physical symptoms include growling stomach, salivating, lack of concentration, feeling light-headed or tired, and thinking about food in the absence of any food cues.

HUNGER EXERCISE

List all the food you ate today. What were your hunger levels when you ate that food, and was it *actual hunger*, *emotional hunger*, or *faux hunger* driving the decision?

_____   _____

_____   _____

_____   _____

_____   _____

_____   _____

_____   _____

- **Emotional hunger:** Sets in suddenly in response to an emotional event. This could be anxiety, sadness, relief at the end of a stressful situation, or even happiness. Emotional hunger demands high-fat and sugary foods. You will not want to eat an apple. Emotional hunger is endless. It will be hard to satisfy.

- **Environmental or faux hunger:** Sets in after seeing, smelling, or talking about food. It can present with physical hunger symptoms, like your mouth watering. It sets in suddenly: if you were not hungry two minutes ago and suddenly you are craving something to eat, you are being driven by your brain and environment—not your stomach.

What you eat throughout the day affects your hunger level, and your diet can be an important reinforcement of your moat. One component of the Target 100 plan (which we'll discuss in more detail in the next chapters) is limiting carbohydrates, in large part because protein and fats keep us fuller longer, and limiting carbs helps us avoid the blood sugar spikes that lead to cravings.

Your Environment at Home

I often make "house calls" to help clients investigate their home environments. I start in the kitchen, but then ask them to walk me through what an average day looks like. Do they end the evening on their couch near the kitchen? Could they move upstairs for the evening to watch TV farther from the call of the fridge? We open every cupboard, and pay close attention to what they see. If they have tempting items in plain sight, each time they see them they will have to confront faux hunger and make a decision not to eat, so we move treats to high, hard-to-reach cupboards.

I can spend hours decluttering and organizing homes, uncovering the ways in which environment is driving overeating, stress, and lack of sleep, exercise, and hydration. I have had more success by helping people move their furniture around to trigger new behaviors than I ever have just by giving someone a meal plan. In my experience, your deeply ingrained habits will trump that meal plan sooner or later. Simply telling yourself you'll stop

Setting up an environment that supports weight loss is actually a set of tasks and habit changes. It requires a good long look around the places where you spend the majority of your time, and, like any other habit change, means investigating possible triggers and creating new ones.

snacking in the evening may not work, but I have seen results improve just by moving side tables away from the couch: when clients go to set their snacks down and find they have nowhere to put them, they remember that they were not supposed to be having a snack in the first place.

Even small changes like entering through the front door instead of a kitchen side door can have a surprising impact. By interrupting her entry routine, a client might suddenly realize that she usually walks in and goes straight to the fridge. I love encouraging clients to start entering through a new door because it further drives home that changing any habit, even such a mundane one, is a real challenge. In fact, they usually won't remember to do it! This reminds them that every change they make must be supported by the habit-loop model. In the case of the client above, she will need to trigger her new entrance route with a reminder—like a sticky note on the door she used to enter through—create a solid new routine by following it repeatedly, and eventually reap the reward of losing weight with less effort because she isn't tempted to snack every time she comes home.

You Are Where You Eat. A study done at Cornell found a link between your weight and the environment in which you eat. Researchers examined "food environments" in the homes of over 200 people and discovered that those who had healthy snack options within sight (like a fruit bowl on a countertop) had lower body weights by up to thirteen pounds. Likewise, those who had unhealthy options—like chips—in sight were up to twenty pounds heavier. Keeping soda around was the worst: it packed on up to twenty-five pounds of extra weight.

Work—The New Food Frontier

The majority of us are now spending more of our waking hours at work—or on the way to and from it—than at home, so it makes sense that I spend just about as much time on my clients' work environments as I do on their environments at home. It would be disastrous to overlook the unique challenges that arise in the office, both in the form of food cues and the stress we often feel in the workplace.

Take a moment to consider what food is available and in plain sight at work. Do you or a coworker have a candy bowl, or snacks stashed in a desk drawer for stressful times? Is there a vending machine or a weekly bagel breakfast that routinely derails your efforts? Do you find that you head to the local deli for lunch with the best of intentions but usually return with an unplanned treat? Investigate your work environment from top to bottom. Remember Rose—even her commute was filled with food cues.

Take a tip from Jennifer and create an environment of health you can bring with you. Consider how the three types of hunger manifest in the work arena. We often underplan for fueling and hydrating ourselves in the workplace. We get overhungry by working through lunch, or eat mindlessly at our desks. Think about how to improve awareness and planning around food, stress, movement, and hydration in your workday.

JENNIFER HUDSON'S PURSE

When I first started working with Jennifer Hudson, she wasn't traveling much and had a fairly regular routine. We set up some healthy habits at home . . . and then her travel schedule picked up like crazy. She struggled with all of the temptations that came along with this, like room service and airport goodies, and we realized that this new normal would force us to think "outside the box" when it came to environment. Jennifer's routine changed every week; it seemed she was never in the same place twice. How could we create habits and consistency for someone who was constantly on the move?

Jennifer loved big, oversized purses, so we began to think of her purse as her moat, a "home" environment that traveled with her. As she prepared for a trip, we made sure that her portable moat was stocked with water, almonds, gum, a banana, individual cheeses, and small bags of popcorn or other single-serve staples like high-quality nutrition bars. Suddenly, we were back on track: Jennifer no longer had to face a myriad of decisions in the stressful environment of an airport, event, or hotel room. She could relax, knowing she had what she needed in her bag to tide her over until she could get a healthy meal.

ENVIRONMENTAL CHANGES EXERCISE

What are three small environmental shifts you could make in the following areas to support weight loss? Check out the Habit Library at the end of this chapter for ideas.

HOME

1. _____
2. _____
3. _____

WORK

1. _____
2. _____
3. _____

SOCIAL SITUATIONS

1. _____
2. _____
3. _____

Keep Your Eyes Open

Work and home are where we spend most of our time, but these days we are exposed to food in so many situations that we need to cultivate environmental awareness everywhere. For example, the average American dines out multiple times a week. Restaurants and malls, movie theaters and sporting events are all food battlefields. Establish this two-part habit to help you avoid overeating or eating when you are not truly hungry:

1. **Think ahead.** Each night before you fall asleep, take five minutes to think through the next day and the food choices you will make. Do you know what you are having for breakfast? What about snacks and lunch? Do

you have a work dinner at a restaurant? If so, take a minute to peruse the menu online to decide what you will eat.

2. **Plan.** Once you have thought through what you will do the next day, you'll need to plan to make it happen. Are you running low on breakfast ingredients? Set a time to get to the store. Do you need ten extra minutes in the morning to make lunch? Set your alarm for ten minutes earlier than usual and place a sticky note on the counter reminding you to make your lunch.

Remember, learning to think ahead and plan is just a habit. Trigger it with a standing appointment in your phone that reminds you to think ahead and plan for the following day. We've mostly talked about our environments in terms of habits involving food, in part because this is where most of the dangers lie, but as you move through the six targets in this book, consider how changes to your environment can support your new habits and prepare you for success in every area of your life.

CHANGE, THE ONLY CONSTANT

Each time something big changes in your life—a new job, a new home, a new relationship—it is an opportunity to start fresh, to train yourself anew. Work to put great habits in place right from the beginning. In smaller ways, too, things are changing around you all the time, and as you grow and transform, you may have to modify your approach. Keep your eyes open for the return or relapse of old habits. Things like a change in season or a shift in responsibilities at work can send routines off course. I recently faced this myself: I'd started to notice that my weight was creeping back up and went into full investigative mode to figure out what was going on. My sons seem to get hungrier by the week, and I realized that not only were they now eating just about every two hours, but my name was their magic wand: "Mom, can I have a snack?" I was confronted with seeing and touching and preparing food many more times each day, and I'd started taking little bites here and there. I strategized a multipronged approach. First, my oldest son was "encouraged" to get his own food. (It's amazing how long you'll keep preparing food for a child who is totally capable of feeding himself!) Second, I created a habit of popping a mint in my mouth whenever I made my youngest a meal or snack, to avoid temptation. These tiny shifts did the trick—but the awareness I needed to make them was the key.

We each have a unique set of habit battles to fight, and the battles never really end. Changing habits can feel like playing whack-a-mole—you get one established, turn your attention to something new . . . and the old habit tries to pop back up. One habit may change easily and without resistance, while another is more complex and requires a longer period of adherence and more vigilant monitoring. It all depends on the depth of the habit, its triggers, and the reward it supplies. The emotions that can accompany habit change are your brain's way of trying to get you to return to the old, comfortable pattern. Remember, old habits are hard to break and new habits are hard to form because the behavioral patterns we repeat are imprinted in our neural pathways. The more you take the road of that new habit, the easier it becomes, but the old road doesn't completely disappear; it is always lurking in the background as a possible path. This is why you may think you have broken an old habit only to find yourself mindlessly repeating it one day out of the blue. It is not a moral failing or a cause for guilt. It is simply a visit to a familiar, friendly pathway that used to get you what you thought you wanted. You *will* relapse into old bad habits. That is not a problem. Success doesn't come from perfection; it comes from recognizing and remedying these slipups more and more quickly. When relapse happens, don't despair—simply pick yourself up and return to the new habit. No guilt or shame; no emotion at all. Just the knowledge that each time you perform that new habit is another solid block in its foundation.

THE MOST IMPORTANT WORKSHEET IN THIS BOOK

I have spent more than fifteen years helping people identify the reasons behind their struggles with weight. When people achieve lasting weight loss, it is because they have dealt with the real issues driving the "food" issues. For example, one client had gotten a great promotion—but no one was hired for the job she vacated. She began essentially filling both roles. This translated into zero time for her to get to the gym, cook healthy food, get to bed on time, or relieve her rapidly mounting stress. It led to resentment, and that led to overeating and drinking because she had no other way to find an "escape." We needed to deal with the job issue first—finding someone to take over the old position and setting up stronger boundaries around work—and then tackle each behavior one at a time. First, get some healthy food in the house, then start getting back to the gym, set a good bedtime routine, reduce drinking. Each one of these is a massive behavior change requiring thought and consideration. Thanks to practice and patience, that client is now well on her way to success.

Before we jump into the targets, the six powerful guidelines you'll tackle using what you've learned in this chapter, I'd like you to tackle the very first worksheet I pull out with every new client I coach. I'm asking you to ask yourself a big question: What is standing in your way? I guarantee it's not that you don't know that eating an apple would be better for you than eating a candy bar! Think for a moment, and identify three big-picture things that are standing in your way. They are likely overarching issues like "not knowing how to say no" or "taking on too much responsibility," "lack of organization," "inability to manage my time," "putting everyone else first," "eating too much sugar," or "not getting enough sleep."

RECOMMENDED READING

The Upward Spiral: Using Neuroscience to Reverse the Course of Depression, One Small Change at a Time, by Alex Korb, PhD

The Power of Habit: Why We Do What We Do in Life and Business, by Charles Duhigg

Mindless Eating: Why We Eat More Than We Think, by Brian Wansink

Once you've identified the three biggest things standing in your way, I want you to pick one of them, and come up with three tasks or behavior changes you could implement this week to address it. Is your problem lack of sleep? This week, set an alarm for thirty minutes before bedtime to begin a routine of turning lights down, screens off, and brushing teeth. Stop using your iPhone as an alarm clock and leave it on the charger at bedtime, so you are not tempted to check email right before you go to sleep. Stop drinking water at a certain time so you don't have to get up in the night to go to the bathroom.

Let me give you two more examples:

- For Sandra, negative self-talk and self-doubt were her greatest obstacles. We set an alarm on her phone to trigger her every morning to track three things she was grateful for, getting positive emotions flowing. We also identified a friend who always made Sandra feel good, and set the task of reaching out to her for support. Finally, Sandra followed three new positive and inspiring wellness accounts on social media so she would see their encouraging messages.

- For Jane, the problem was lack of time to make and eat healthy meals. We set up a twice-weekly meal-delivery service for her, covering four meals and ordering twice as much as she needed to help her with healthier lunches for work as well. She was also tasked with buying new Tupperware and a nice cooler bag to take lunch in. Jane set aside a half hour in her work calendar every day to sit in the cafeteria and eat, away from her desk and the distraction of work, which had often led to her skipping lunch and getting overhungry by dinnertime.

Now it is your turn. Fill out the worksheet below—really consider what will have the greatest impact right now. Then, using this worksheet and the Habit Change Key from earlier in the chapter, make a plan. Face this one issue, take three small steps, and watch your life change, one habit at a time.

BEHAVIOR MODIFICATION WORKSHEET

CHALLENGES:

What are the three biggest things standing in the way of your progress? *(Examples—Not enough time, putting everyone else first, lack of knowledge, lack of preparation, organization . . .)*

1. _____

2. _____

3. _____

Which of these three things will you work on this week?

_____

TASKS/BEHAVIOR CHANGES:

Write out three small tasks or behavior changes, related to the issue you have chosen, that you will tackle this week to begin breaking down the challenge. *(Examples—This week I will . . . grocery shop on Sunday, get up fifteen minutes earlier to make lunch, plan dinners . . .)*

1. _____

2. _____

3. _____

REWARD:
Decide how you will reward yourself for a job well done!
(Examples—new running shoes, go to a movie, get a massage . . .)

_____

HABIT LIBRARY

The following are twenty-five of the most common habits and tasks my clients have found helpful, especially in addressing their environment. You will notice a Habit Library at the end of each chapter, geared to that chapter's topic. Use these libraries as a place to begin brainstorming about what personal habits you might want to change or cultivate, and feel free to borrow from them.

1. Take a minute before and after a meal to notice your hunger level and how you feel.
2. Drink a big glass of water as soon as you wake up.
3. Track one meal in a food journal.
4. Get to bed thirty minutes earlier.
5. Drink water with each meal.
6. Clean your kitchen.
7. Place treats out of sight.
8. Stop eating after dinner.
9. Chew mint gum while grocery shopping.
10. Carry healthy snacks with you in your bag, purse, briefcase, or backpack.
11. Turn off all screens during meals.
12. Before you go out to eat, look up the menu and think about what you might choose.
13. Clean the fridge.
14. Rearrange the furniture in the room where you are most often tempted to snack.
15. Sit in a new location for your nighttime relaxation or TV time.
16. Put leftovers away before sitting down to dinner.
17. Stop serving dinner "family style" at the table—instead, plate food before you sit.
18. Place a food scale on the counter where you can see it and get to it easily.
19. Begin brushing your teeth right after dinner.
20. Set alarms for meal and snack times so you do not get overhungry at work.
21. Start packing a lunch instead of buying it.
22. Stock a drawer at work with healthy staples for times when hunger hits.
23. Replace screens with books after a certain point in the evening to cut down on food cues.
24. Get in the habit of grocery shopping right after a meal so that you aren't hungry while you shop.
25. Stop eating lunch at your desk.

Chapter 2

INTRODUCING THE SIX TARGETS

O n vacation a few years ago, I signed up for an afternoon of archery with my sons. We decided to make it a friendly competition, but when I raised my (surprisingly heavy!) bow and looked toward the target, I found myself thinking that the yellow bull's-eye looked *awfully* tiny. *This is going to be impossible*, I thought to myself. But here's the thing: even though a bull's-eye will get you the most points, you also get points when the arrow lands outside it, in one of the target's other circles. Over the course of the afternoon I never did get a bull's-eye, but not only did I steadily improve my aim, I racked up a pretty impressive score just by being consistently imperfect. Several not–bull's-eyes are worth a lot more than a single bull's-eye, and my score was certainly higher than it would have been if I had tried once, decided not hitting the center meant failure, and given up.

The imagery of that archery target is what guided me as I created this program. What I see all too often in my clients (and in myself) is a self-defeating perfectionism, a belief that we must hit the bull's-eye every time we eat a meal, go to the gym, or step on the scale. When we fall short of our punishing expectations, we often give up for the day or for good, frustrated and feeling hopeless. In weight loss, however, consistency beats perfection every time.

SIX TARGETS, ONE NUMBER, ZERO PUNISHMENT

Target 100 is a holistic program based on the premise that absolutism doesn't work in weight loss. Instead, it shows you how to make small, meaningful adjustments that will lead to permanent behavior change and successful, long-term weight loss. Target 100 is the product of everything I have learned over the course of my career: every focus group, every interview, every private client, every personal experience. It draws on the latest research in fields like nutrition, exercise, mindfulness, sleep, and habit science. I wanted the program to be simple but effective, flexible enough to fit into any lifestyle. After a lot of experimentation and trial and error, I settled on six doable, easy-to-remember guidelines that, combined, produce dramatic results. Each addresses a different piece of the weight-loss puzzle, and each sets a "target" of 100:

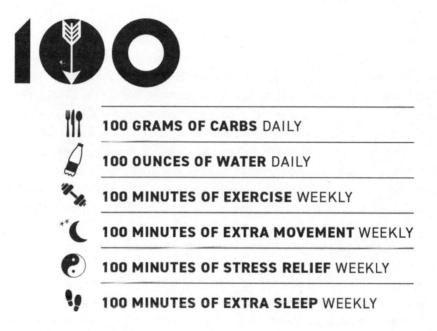

100 GRAMS OF CARBS DAILY

100 OUNCES OF WATER DAILY

100 MINUTES OF EXERCISE WEEKLY

100 MINUTES OF EXTRA MOVEMENT WEEKLY

100 MINUTES OF STRESS RELIEF WEEKLY

100 MINUTES OF EXTRA SLEEP WEEKLY

For each of these guidelines, 100 is the goal—the yellow bull's-eye in the center of the target—but just as in archery, it isn't all or nothing. If you can't add 100 minutes of sleep per week, you will still make progress by adding eighty minutes, sixty minutes, or even forty minutes. All of your efforts "count" and will produce results as long as you keep *making* that effort—perfection is *not* a prerequisite for weight loss.

This is where I beg you to trust me. I can feel your skepticism because I see it in almost every client. Everyone thinks that weight loss has to hurt to work. "No pain, no gain," right? We have lost the weight, gained it back, tried to lose it again so many times in such punishing ways, it is hard to believe that small, deliberate lifestyle changes will be more effective than any crash diet you've ever tried. I've become an expert on what works—and what doesn't—to achieve weight-loss success, not only by losing weight myself but by helping scores of others lose the weight and keep it off, and success didn't come in the form of extreme restriction or a rigid regimen for a single one of them. The solution itself was never extraordinary, even when it delivered extraordinary results. Every time, success came from sustainable, personalized changes, building a solid foundation of healthy habits.

THE SENSE BEHIND THE SIX

Why *these* targets? And are they all really that important? The answers to these questions will be addressed in much more detail later, in the chapters devoted to each target (spoiler alert—the answer to the second question is *yes!*), but for now, let me begin with the fact that the truth about weight loss is much more complex than we have been admitting. We want to believe the weight-loss equation is as simple as calories in and calories out, but ignoring the other variables doesn't make them disappear. Diet is a big part of the picture, but as we discussed in the previous chapter, no meal plan will save you from your habits. We are being triggered and faced with food decisions at every turn—over 200 per day—while newly created foods are engineered to be addictive. Lack of hydration is driving us to overeat and sapping our energy. Endless low-level stressors are flooding us with hormones that drive our decisions and alter the way we process fat. Exercise has become tangled with food, something we view as a punishment or a get-out-of-jail-free card, weighed down with shame and unrealistic expectations. Our increasingly sedentary lives are stifling our metabolisms and changing the way our bodies function. Lack of sleep exhausts our reserves and increases levels of the hormones that tell us to eat, while cutting production of those that tell us when to stop. These examples only scratch the surface, but they should be enough to make it clear that we won't get far with good intentions and calorie counting.

But as complex as the weight-loss equation is, the solution doesn't have to be complicated—in fact, to work, the solution *must* be a simple one. After so many years in the weight-loss industry, one thing I know to be true is that no one feels like decoding and demystifying a complicated weight-loss program. Taking weight off in our environment is hard enough without lists of requirements to memorize and demanding hoops to jump through. When people abandon their efforts to lose weight or get healthy, they often cite feeling too busy and overwhelmed to stay on top of all the components of their chosen plan. After all, our lives are about so much more than losing weight. We are working longer hours, raising families, taking care of parents, going back to school, and more. We don't have time for weight-loss programs that are like working a second job—some of us already have second jobs! Target 100 doesn't ask you to count every gram of every nutrient and every calorie you eat at every meal, or to arrange your life around your weight loss, but it is transformative just the same. This simple plan works so well because each of the six targets has wide-ranging impact. For example:

- When you limit yourself to 100 grams of carbs each day, you don't have to bother counting calories, or grams of protein or fat—these fall into place by default. You naturally increase your consumption of proteins, fats, and filling vegetables, and reduce your consumption of sugar and processed foods. Blood sugar levels out, keeping your energy on a steady keel, and you are released from the cycle of cravings. The foods you eat are more satisfying and keep you fuller longer, making it easier to avoid temptation.

- When you drink 100 ounces of water each day, you avoid the call to eat sent out by a dehydrated body attempting to find water in food. You keep your metabolism humming and your digestion running smoothly. You are less hungry, think more clearly, and have more energy.

- When you get 100 minutes of exercise each week, you unlearn the lessons of past failures, and see instead that you are strong and capable. You train

Achieving successful, lasting weight loss is like building a house, or keeping a circus tent aloft, or playing a game of Jenga— go ahead, pick your metaphor! The formula for habit change is your foundation; and stress, sleep, hydration, nutrition, exercise, and movement are all vital structural elements, braced by and supporting each other. Overlook or weaken any one of them and the whole thing could topple over.

your mind as you train your body, gaining the power to push through discomfort while building lean muscle and burning fat.

- When you add 100 minutes of movement to your week, you gain momentum and energy, kick-starting your metabolism and creating the habits that support long-term health and weight maintenance while fighting disease.
- When you get 100 minutes of stress relief each week, you neutralize the powerful hormonal maelstrom of stress. You give yourself the emotional and physical resilience you need to stay committed to your goals and make better choices in every area of your life.
- When you add 100 minutes of sleep to your week, you have the energy and stamina you need to succeed. You refresh your body, and help stabilize the action of hormones that regulate appetite, satiety, and metabolism.

As you read about and take action on each of these targets, you will begin to see that they all support one another; that each makes the others easier. Targeting 100 minutes of exercise will reduce stress, help you sleep better at night, build confidence, and combat negative thoughts. Those effects will in turn make it easier to make better food choices. The reduction of carbs will reduce inflammation and sugar crashes, making it easier to get and stay moving, while the increase in protein helps you maintain and build lean muscle. Drinking 100 ounces of water each day supports the activity of exercise and helps the body recover, while being active in the first place triggers you to drink the water your body needs. I could go on, but I think you get the idea.

ANATOMY OF A SUCCESS STORY

We pick up the idea that weight loss is something magical from the advertising we see. I used to marvel at the beautiful posters hanging in Weight Watchers centers across the country. Sad-faced, slump-shouldered "Before" photos juxtaposed with a smiling, laughing, windblown "After."

before

JANUARY
15

MARCH
20

APRIL
5

JUNE
30

after

Putting the two photos right next to each other removes all that happened in between: all the tiny changes and new habits, the days of frustration, the moments of wanting to quit but sticking it out.

Don't be fooled into thinking that there is a magic formula, program, or pill that will change your life *for* you. At the same time, any single thing you want to change or habit you want to build is within your reach, by examining what is involved and taking small, methodical steps toward your goal. This is the common thread in every weight-loss success story: arriving at a place where you understand that consistent, enjoyable progress forward, no matter how slow, offers more than any quick change ever can.

Below is what I *wish* you could see in a before and after photo.

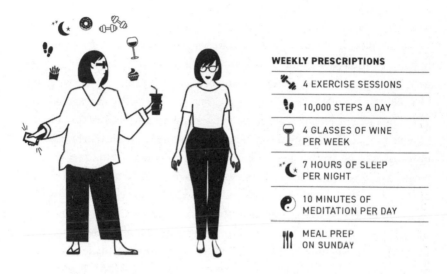

WEEKLY PRESCRIPTIONS

4 EXERCISE SESSIONS

10,000 STEPS A DAY

4 GLASSES OF WINE
PER WEEK

7 HOURS OF SLEEP
PER NIGHT

10 MINUTES OF
MEDITATION PER DAY

MEAL PREP
ON SUNDAY

BEFORE:

Dehydrated, drinking mostly diet soda, rarely cooking, eating mostly processed foods, not exercising, most days spent sitting, getting fewer than 5,000 steps per day, dessert and two alcoholic beverages every night, skipping lunch, getting overhungry (and then overeating as a result), watching TV to fall asleep at night, sleep deprived, constantly checking work email even on weekends, stressed-out and overwhelmed.

AFTER:

Walking to and from work, placing three water bottles strategically to trigger hydration, having groceries delivered weekly, bringing lunch to work, cooking three nights a week, drinking less alcohol, eating a protein-filled breakfast, exercising four times a week, recharging with a weekly yoga class or by meeting a friend for a walk, spending less time on the phone and checking email only at scheduled times, getting a solid seven hours of sleep each night.

DIRECTION, NOT DEMANDS

Typical weight-loss books give orders: Eat this, don't eat that; do this, don't do that. That works for some people, especially for short periods of time. But seven days, two weeks, or thirty days are only a blink of an eye when compared to how long we live. The result is familiar to most of us—finishing a month-long diet "challenge" only to slide inevitably back to old habits and behaviors. This is why Target 100 is about more than the targets themselves: the program is powered by the engine of habit change, which we will return to in every chapter. Talking about one without the other—giving guidelines without guidance—will never work.

Target 100 aims to be the last program you ever follow, and it can succeed in part because you will not really be following, you will be leading your own way. This is the other key difference between Target 100 and typical weight-loss programs: it offers flexibility, not rigidity, because as I've said again and again, no one-size-fits-all plan can possibly know what will work for you or what particular challenges you face. I will outline the basic tenets and give you the tools to change your behavior, but you must begin to trust that you and only you know which habits and behaviors are standing in the way of your success, and which changes will enable it. No one can make those decisions for you. By following Target 100's six guidelines, you'll naturally move toward permanent weight loss by eating more whole foods and cutting down on sugar, keeping your body hydrated, increasing activity levels, reducing stress, and sleeping better—but the particulars of those behaviors will be largely up to you.

The weight-loss process can be overwhelming when you look at all of the changes you will eventually have to make; in an effort to simplify this, I have laid out a ten-week "plan" following this chapter. In truth, Target 100 is plan agnostic. Maybe you have a food plan or an exercise practice that works well for you already—that's great! Feel free to layer Target 100's principles on top of whatever you are doing. The suggested ten-week outline simply gives you a structured way to implement these principles. Its most important function is to drive home the point that you are *not* meant to tackle the six targets all at once on day one. I've **found that clients see the most success when they tackle one target at a time.** In fact, for the very first week, I focus not just on one target, but on one meal: breakfast. After that, I have placed targets in the sequence that seems to resonate most with clients—after years of approaching weight loss from a food perspective, they seem to "need" to start by tackling food and water. We then quickly move to movement, exercise, stress, and sleep. You can opt to dissect this plan and do it in any order you wish, or you can ignore it altogether. You can read the rest of the book all at once, or move through it chapter by chapter. I have given you every tip and resource I have at my disposal. After the chapters on the individual targets, you'll find a chapter on support and another on technology—two crucial resources you should absolutely take advantage of. I've also included a section of ten of my favorite recipes that are low in carbs and in effort.

By the end of this book, you will have created your very own formula for success. Yours will be completely unique and totally personal, based upon what *you* like to eat, how *you* like to move, and what *your* life actually looks like. Do you need three workouts a week or five? Do you feel best with six mini-meals or three squares a day? What are your most effective triggers, your most effective ways to combat stress? That formula will always be yours; no one will be able to take it from you. Should you fall away from healthy habits for a time, it will be there when you return, and it will grow and change along with you as old challenges disappear and new ones arise.

After you've tackled each target for the first time over the course of a number of weeks, you will *keep* tackling each of the six pillars, just as we all do every day as we make decisions about wellness, whether intentionally or not. You will learn to decode for yourself if you need to focus on a slipping hydration habit or challenging yourself to add exercise minutes or packing lunches to take to work. The Habit Libraries at the end of each chapter are full of suggestions to aid you in brainstorming concrete ways to address whatever you are working on, but be creative and enjoy the process of growth. Eventually, Target 100 makes itself obsolete. Once you integrate its principles into your life, you'll find you are no longer following a program, you are simply living with awareness and balance, using what you've learned about yourself to build the life you want. You are free.

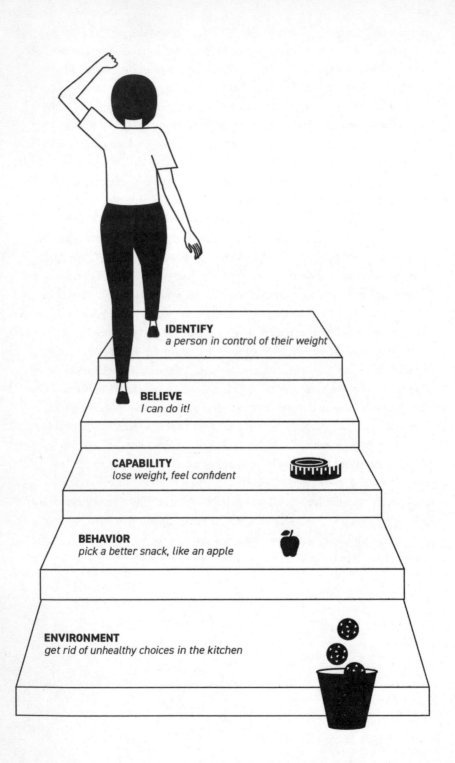

IDENTIFY
a person in control of their weight

BELIEVE
I can do it!

CAPABILITY
lose weight, feel confident

BEHAVIOR
pick a better snack, like an apple

ENVIRONMENT
get rid of unhealthy choices in the kitchen

Taking Aim

YOUR TEN-WEEK PLAN

ABOUT THIS PLAN

Little libraries: For each week's topic, I have included a list of the five habits and tasks that have given clients the greatest success. There are another twenty in the full Habit Library for each chapter, but these five can be an easy jumping-off point if you're feeling overwhelmed.

Tracking success: I am suggesting that you weigh in at least once a week—and certainly right at the beginning. If possible, use a scale that measures body fat so you can see progress (particularly as you add exercise) even on weeks in which your weight doesn't reflect it. Reframe the relationship you have with your scale: a scale is a tool and a guide, *not* a tyrant deciding your fate. Track your weight in an app or a notebook so that you can see your progress over time. Additionally, I ask my clients to track the habits they change. Being able to look back on all the behaviors you've battled and transformed will help you understand that the scale is not the only measure of success.

Don't forget your secret weapon: When I was trying every weight-loss fad under the sun, I often bought a diet book and skipped right to the "plan" or better yet, the "quick start" section and started there. If you are tempted to do the same . . . *don't*. Chapter One was the longest chapter in this book for good reason—it is also the most important. It gives you the tools that power this program. It is absolutely not optional. If you skipped it, go back to it now. Take the time to do the exercises, complete the worksheet at the end, and spend a week doing the work it asks of you. You won't regret it.

WEEK ONE: BEGIN WITH BREAKFAST

Weigh in

Read—or reread—Chapter Three: Beginning with Breakfast

Target 100 is all about the transformative power of small steps. I love spending our first week on breakfast because it requires enough planning and habit change to be a challenge, while also remaining simple enough to feel manageable and give you a motivating taste of success. It is a perfect way to drive home the fact that small changes can have outsized effects: it gets you off to a healthy start right away in the morning (often leading to better choices all day), and by shifting to a lower-carb breakfast, you will feel less hunger and fewer cravings later on.

Top Habits and Tasks:
1. Set your alarm fifteen to thirty minutes early each morning to allow time to prep and eat your breakfast.
2. Brainstorm your five favorite easy breakfasts. Leave the list where you can see it in the kitchen.
3. Stock up on breakfast ingredients and grab-and-go options.
4. Try using leftovers for breakfast.
5. Decide where you will eat breakfast and make sure the space is clear and clean before you go to bed each night.

WEEK TWO: TARGET 100 GRAMS OF CARBS

Weigh in

Read—or reread—Chapter Four: Food That Fuels

This week is all about expanding upon the skills you developed by perfecting your breakfast, and beginning to understand what it looks like to stay below 100 grams of carbs for the day. Take the time to fill out the 5-5-5 Worksheet, creating favorite meals that are easy and help you stay on track. For ideas, try the recipes at the end of this book or search the internet for "low-carb meals." Use an app or a notebook to track your carbs each day, especially in this first week, to ensure that you are coming in around 100 grams. You may want to experiment with different sizes of meals and snacks, noting how you feel throughout the day.

<u>**Top Habits and Tasks:**</u>

1. Schedule a specific time for weekly meal planning and to stock up on anything you need.
2. Add a fruit or vegetable to every meal or snack.
3. Carry healthy snacks with you in your bag or purse.
4. Double the recipe for a healthy meal and use the leftovers over the next few days.
5. Try grocery delivery to avoid the temptation of the grocery store.

WEEK THREE: TARGET 100 OUNCES OF WATER

Weigh in

Read—or reread—Chapter Five: Water, Water, Everywhere

Now that you are beginning to get a handle on food, this week is all about layering the habit of hydration on top of keeping your carbs around 100 grams. Tracking your ounces doesn't have to be hard: if you have a big thirty-two-ounce tumbler, for instance, just make sure you drink three of these. Notice how much more satisfied you feel and how your energy perks up—and how much easier your food choices are becoming.

<u>**Top Habits and Tasks:**</u>

1. Drink one full glass of water upon waking.
2. Get a new water bottle or tumbler to keep with you.
3. Set alarms on your phone to remind you to drink water at set points throughout the day.
4. Drink a full glass of water before each meal.
5. Use the habit loop to drop soda—regular *and* diet—completely.

WEEK FOUR: TARGET 100 MINUTES OF EXERCISE

Weigh in

Read—or reread—Chapter Six: Exercise Therapy

This week you begin training your brain with exercise, building your confidence and your strength, both mental and physical. Adding exercise to your budding food and water habits may seem like a lot of plates to keep spinning, but each practice should make the others easier and build momentum. Your 100 minutes can be divided any way you like, and it may change week to week: Take a sixty-minute class and do a forty-minute DVD, or schedule three thirty-five-minute workouts at the gym. If you find skipping days makes it hard to jump back in, especially at first, try a week where you exercise every day, but for just fifteen minutes. Find what works for you—and remember to start where you are! If you are starting from zero, you don't have to leap to 100 minutes all at once: try twenty minutes a week and work upward from there.

Top Habits and Tasks:

1. Set out your workout clothes at night to trigger you to exercise in the morning.
2. Ask a friend to meet you for a workout or a run.
3. Buy a new pair of shoes for your new exercise habit.
4. Schedule your exercise sessions one week ahead.
5. Research exercise classes in your neighborhood.

WEEK FIVE: TARGET BOREDOM— NEW DISCOVERY WEEK

Weigh in

This week you aren't going to tackle a new target. Keep up with your carbs, your water, and your exercise . . . and try at least three new meals and one new workout.

It's not widely known to the general public, but those of us who have worked in weight loss for many years have learned that, after about four weeks, new dieters and fitness converts reach an exhaustion point. Many give up then, because they don't realize it is "normal" to get bored and lose focus at this stage—I make sure clients are aware of the four-week slump and have a plan in place to combat boredom and fatigue. This is an additional skill that will improve your chances of long-term success. We all get stuck in ruts. This week, set aside time to roam the internet for new recipes, check out streaming offerings or a local dance studio, and just generally make an effort to keep things fresh.

Top Habits and Tasks:

1. Set an appointment with yourself, for the same time each week, to look for new recipes.

2. Ask a friend to try a new fitness class with you—make it an adventure!
3. Try a fruit or vegetable that you have never eaten before.
4. If you usually exercise in the morning, try exercising in the evening, or vice versa.
5. Have breakfast for dinner or dinner for breakfast.

WEEK SIX: TARGET 100 MINUTES OF MOVEMENT

Weigh in

Read—or reread—Chapter Seven: Move More

Hopefully, you are feeling refreshed from your week of boredom busting and ready to take on your next target: movement. Add 100 minutes to your movement baseline this week, and notice how moving more makes it easier to keep moving. You can get your 100 minutes by adding walks, but also by cleaning the house, gardening, dancing while you cook dinner, or playing outside with the kids.

Top Habits and Tasks:
1. Set alarms to remind you to get up every thirty minutes (or use a wearable device that vibrates to remind you to move when you've been sedentary too long).
2. Add walking to your commute.
3. Ask a friend to join you for a walk.
4. Get a wearable device, pedometer, or app that counts steps on your phone.
5. Take a fifteen-minute walk after dinner.

WEEK SEVEN: TARGET 100 MINUTES OF STRESS REDUCTION

Weigh in

Read—or reread—Chapter Eight: Stress Less

Now that we know how our stress levels are affecting our weight and driving our decisions, it's time to target stress reduction. You can split these 100 minutes up any way you like, and, as always, feel free to change things up from week to week. You may choose to spend forty minutes journaling each Saturday, and knock out the remaining sixty minutes with five fifteen-minute meditation sessions one week, and a mindful walk and a bubble bath the next. It's up to you! Seek out and practice simple stress-relief techniques you can use throughout your day, whenever you feel stress building, to halt the body's flood of adrenaline and cortisol.

Top Habits and Tasks:

1. Download a meditation app.
2. Practice deep breathing.
3. Stop using the snooze button.
4. Stop checking work email once you are finished with work for the evening!
5. Take a ten-minute walk outside at the peak stress time of your day.

WEEK EIGHT: TARGET 100 MINUTES OF SLEEP

Weigh in

Read—or reread—Chapter Nine: Sleep Your Way to Success

Sleep is your body's essential recovery time. Without it, you will battle fatigue and sluggishness, alongside wild hormone swings that hound you to eat. Create conditions that support quality sleep. Examine your bedtime routine, and allow yourself to wind down at night. Begin to play around with the amount of sleep you get to discover your perfect amount—and then work to protect it and ensure you are getting that amount regularly. You can get your 100 extra minutes in no time by getting to sleep just fifteen minutes earlier.

Top Habits and Tasks:

1. Begin dimming lights two hours before bedtime.
2. Set an alarm for thirty minutes before you want to be in bed to remind you to start getting ready.
3. Ban screens from the bedroom.
4. Stop using a smartphone as an alarm so you are not tempted to browse the web at night or first thing in the morning.
5. Read before bed instead of watching TV.

WEEK NINE: TARGET YOUR TOOLBOX

Weigh in
Read—or reread—Chapters Ten and Eleven: You Need a Network, and
Technology Is Your Friend

When you have a strong support network, you turn environment from an enemy to an ally. Technology provides us with much-needed triggers and endlessly evolving tools, all while expanding our support system. Set aside this week to find ways to use support and technology to make your life and your program easier and more livable. Try a meal-box delivery service, enlist a friend in your weight-loss challenge, join a recipe-sharing group on Facebook, or download a habit-building app to help trigger and keep track of the new behaviors you are working on.

Top Habits and Tasks:
1. Try a meal delivery service.
2. Sign up for a fitness class where you'll see the same people each week—and maybe make some new friends.
3. Tell friends about your goals.
4. Set aside twenty minutes for exploring apps or scrolling through recipe or weight-loss sites for inspiration and motivation.
5. Join the Target 100 Facebook group for support.

WEEK TEN: TAKE IT UP A NOTCH

Weigh in

Now it is time to see how this is done over the long haul. The series of new behaviors and habits that you've set up throughout the past nine weeks will begin to feel more natural. You're hydrated, getting to bed on time, relieving stress, eating better, moving more, and even working out. Yay you! Now it is time to revisit the targets systematically to observe where you are—what needs work and how you might push yourself one step further. This week, take a moment to focus on each of the six targets and implement one small change in each area to advance your progress. For example, maybe you have been getting to bed on time but know that your sleep environment could really use a makeover. Set aside a two-hour chunk of time to rearrange the furniture and remove the old TV from your bedroom. Maybe get some new sheets and clear clutter from your sleep space. This will make your new habit of getting the right amount of sleep even stronger. You will begin to look forward to getting into bed and associate your bedroom with restful peace. Now take a look at the other five pillars and set a tiny goal within each one, like getting a few new songs on your workout playlist, adding a new snack into your snack rotation, making sure you are hydrating evenly throughout the day, and so on.

This is how a healthy lifestyle grows. You simply look ahead at your week and decide on one new action to propel you forward. If you're struggling in a certain area, maybe you don't add anything new, but instead refocus your efforts where they're needed. Use your habit loop and any of the worksheets that I have supplied. Make copies and use them to periodically reexamine and rework your plan. Watch out for old habits that are cropping back up and changes that demand new ones. Stay conscious and aware, talk to yourself kindly and without guilt or shame, and build trust and confidence by keeping your promises to yourself. Most of all, enjoy seeing yourself transform, and relish the empowerment that comes of knowing that *your life is yours to change.*

Top Habits and Tasks:

1. **Food.** Try a new recipe.
2. **Water.** Drop a nonwater drink from your day (soda, coffee, or alcohol) and replace with water.
3. **Exercise.** Add five extra minutes to your workout.
4. **Movement.** Add 1,000 extra steps or ten extra minutes of walking to your day.
5. **Stress.** Try a new type of meditation.
6. **Sleep.** Clean up your sleep environment.

TARGETS
1 AND 2

FOOD AND WATER

Chapter 3

BEGINNING WITH BREAKFAST

I ran into Becky, a neighbor of mine, in the grocery store a while back and was astonished by the mountain of food she was buying. I have two sons and a very active husband, so, believe me, I'm no stranger to huge grocery runs. But Becky's cart was so full that I don't think she could have fit one more thing in—it was loaded up in a way that defied gravity.

"I'm starting a new diet," Becky explained when she noticed me eyeing her cart. "This morning I got rid of all the bad food in the house, and now I'm restocking." She showed me her new diet's recommended grocery list, which had at least a hundred items on it, from agave to zucchini.

"I just wish I liked plain Greek yogurt," Becky said, making a face as she pointed to a pile of yogurt containers. "I hate the way it tastes, but I have to have it every day in this Super Breakfast Smoothie. I'm hoping the kale and the avocado cover up the taste of the yogurt." Judging from the face she made, I got the definite impression that kale and avocado weren't big favorites either.

As we chatted, I learned that in addition to restocking her kitchen with trips to the supermarket and specialty food stores that day, Becky planned to head over to the local gym to sign up for a membership and run to the mall to buy a twelve-quart stockpot (for making bone broth??) and a spiral slicer (to cut veggies into pasta shapes). At least all of her running around would have a side benefit: "I have to put in ten thousand steps," she said, pointing to a brand-new counter on her wrist. Becky headed toward the checkout lanes, and I wished her luck. "I hope this works," she confided. "I've only been following this plan for four hours, and I'm already exhausted!"

I hoped so, too, but in all honestly, I had little faith that it would. Maybe you think I should have told Becky as much, but as a weight-loss coach, I know many of my friends already turn and run when they see me at a restaurant or a grocery store for fear I'll judge their choices, and I've learned not to give unsolicited advice. But Becky's new program, with its all-or-nothing approach and its inflexible list of do-this, don't-do-that requirements, reminded me of so many other one-size-fits-all diets that I've seen fail over the years. I wasn't at all surprised when I saw Becky again a couple of months later, having abandoned the diet and feeling worse about herself than before.

Most of my clients come to me like Becky, post-diet—full of regret at a long line of perceived failures and secretly feeling that nothing will ever work. It's hard for me to see anyone this way, friend or stranger, maybe because this was *me* for so many years. And if this sounds like you, I want you to understand that you have nothing to be ashamed of. You are *not* a failure. In fact, you are my hero. You have stepped into the ring over and over to face a powerful opponent. You've kept trying, and if you haven't succeeded, it is simply because you were never given the training you needed.

A BETTER WAY

The problem with diet plans like Becky's is that they demand way, way too much of their followers. They expect you to empty out your kitchen, buy hundreds of dollars' worth of new groceries and gadgets, force yourself to live on certain foods whether you like them or not, jump into unfamiliar fitness programs, become a teetotaler, and make a monk-like commitment to *their* vision . . . oh and by the way, they want you to do it all at once.

In other words, they demand that you commit 100 percent to a plan that was designed by people you've never met, who have absolutely no awareness of your personal tastes, preferences, background, or lifestyle.

My weight-loss approach is 180 degrees from the rigid, my-way-or-the-highway diet path. I won't tell you to get rid of a dumpster full of food. I won't tell you to plunge into an extreme exercise regimen or invest in expensive appliances you'll use once or twice. And I certainly won't tell you to make a hundred major life changes all in one day. Yeah, you need to make some adjustments to how you eat and move—you wouldn't have cracked open this book if you didn't have some ineffective habits and behaviors. But you don't have to—and simply *shouldn't*—make these changes all at the same time!

In fact, we're going to start with just one thing: breakfast.

Why breakfast? Because it's the easiest place to start. And because the wisdom you gain as you rethink that first meal will support and guide you as you face the hundreds of food choices that confront you each day. Beginning with breakfast is like a new runner starting by jogging around her block rather than trying to run a marathon her first day out. From this point on, let breakfast serve as a metaphor. Let it stand for the small, measured, incremental—and, above all, *livable*—changes you make on the way to transforming your life for good.

Reinventing your breakfast not only teaches you the skills you'll need when addressing your diet as a whole, it opens your eyes to the intricacies of making any single change. For example, as you develop your breakfast strategy, here are just a few of the things you'll have to consider:

- What foods will you need to have on hand for breakfast?
- When will you shop for them?
- Where will you eat breakfast—at the kitchen table, in your car, at your desk at work?
- Will you prepare your breakfast in the morning, or get it ready the night before?
- Will your breakfast plan affect what time you get up in the morning?
- If you exercise in the morning, will you eat breakfast before or after your workout?
- Will your breakfast choices differ on your workout days?
- How will breakfast fit in with your other morning tasks, such as feeding your kids, making lunches, getting ready for work, and so on?

All of these decisions—and this is by no means an exhaustive list—go into changing *just one meal*. You can see why diets that have you attacking everything at once are so prone to failure—there isn't a chance you will manage all those changes without an immense amount of stress and discomfort. Every meal has its own challenges and choices, but by working first on the decisions and behaviors surrounding breakfast, you can begin to identify strategies and preferences that will work for other meals as well.

As a bonus, here's something I've noticed about breakfast: When people get their breakfast on track, they often start to lose weight even without making deliberate changes to *any other meal*. Breakfast makes up a third of your meals for the day, so if you alter your intake there, it makes sense that you will experience some weight loss with only that change. But the more important reason clients see results just from adjusting their breakfast is that this one meal fuels us physically and emotionally in a way that inspires us to make better choices throughout the day, both consciously and unconsciously. Breakfast is the first meal of the day—but, symbolically, it's so much more: It's a new beginning, a clean slate, a fresh opportunity. Designing a truly personalized breakfast strategy sets you on the path to long-term weight loss without overwhelming you, and it gives you a way to experience some success right away. Once you master breakfast, you'll be motivated and ready to tackle other difficult behaviors.

FIVE STEPS TO A BETTER BREAKFAST

The goal of reinventing breakfast is to figure out how to make this meal work for *you*. After giving it some thought, you may decide that your current breakfast strategy is just right, requiring no changes at all. Or you may realize that some adjustments, large or small, are definitely in order. Either way, the purpose of this chapter is to discover what will serve you best in terms of nutrition, energy, and impact on food cravings and hunger later in the day. You'll also consider your food preferences, current habits, and schedule. Then we'll create a customized breakfast plan that will start your day off right and help you reach your weight-loss goals.

Step 1: Examine Your Assumptions

You've probably heard it a million times: "Breakfast is the most important meal of the day." There is so much conventional wisdom about what to eat, how much to eat, and indeed, *whether* to eat breakfast. The problem with all these standard beliefs about breakfast is that they're not necessarily true. There is no perfect breakfast that works for everyone. The reality is, the best breakfast for *you* may not be the best breakfast for *me*. And for some, the best breakfast may even be no breakfast at all.

Once you figure out what your best breakfast is like, you can stop following everyone else's advice about what you *should* and *should not* eat in the morning and choose a meal that will give you what you need. As I look back at my own weight-loss journey, I am reminded that I went from consuming nothing but Diet Coke in the morning to eating well-balanced, low-calorie breakfasts, to now eating a larger, much lower-carbohydrate meal higher in fats and proteins to keep me satisfied. It has been a journey from one thing to the next, requiring exploration and trial and error.

Some of my clients do best with a big breakfast. They wake up starving, and a good-sized meal energizes them. Without it, they feel lethargic and hungry all day. When they follow diet plans that recommend small breakfasts, they trudge moodily through the hours, feeling deprived and lacking energy. Lunch fails to inspire them, and by midafternoon they

There's been some dispute over whether it's OK to skip breakfast. For a long time, people have believed that going without breakfast inevitably leads to overeating later in the day. On the other hand, some weight-loss experts actually recommend skipping breakfast. Who is correct?

I've taken a good look at the research, and I've found that the results are quite mixed. Some studies find a modest weight-loss benefit for people who eat breakfast; others find no benefit at all. The same is true with skipping breakfast—some studies suggest it helps with weight loss, and others find it has no effect. Skipping breakfast is a form of intermittent fasting, a weight-loss strategy that has become popular lately. But like all such strategies, it doesn't work for everyone.

What all these studies and their varying results tell me is that when it comes to breakfast, like most everything else, the best path to weight-loss success is figuring out what works for you—and then doing it.

find themselves sneaking chocolate or reaching for chips. A small breakfast seems to destine them to a day of growling stomachs and dissatisfaction.

Other clients have done best with small breakfasts—or no breakfast at all. When they wake up they have little or no hunger, and it barely occurs to them to eat a meal. When they follow diet plans that demand a big breakfast, these people force-feed themselves a meal they'd be just as happy without. Eating so much in the morning leaves them stuffed and listless for hours. Worse, it sometimes triggers midmorning hunger that they wouldn't feel if they hadn't had breakfast in the first place.

I've seen too many people force themselves to eat breakfast because it's what they believe they *should* do, even though it makes them nauseated and hungrier later in the day. I've also seen too many people who want a hearty bacon-and-egg type of meal try to make do with yogurt or a smoothie even though it causes their blood sugar to crash or makes them headachy and irritable. This is madness! When these people listen to their bodies, make the food choices that fit *them*, and build new breakfast habits that support these choices, they typically feel better, more energetic, and more focused throughout the day. And they usually start having a lot more luck losing weight.

To sum up, we hold a lot of unquestioned beliefs about what constitutes a "good" breakfast. This first step is all about making the decision to let them go.

Step 2: Think Outside the Cereal Box

Eggs and bacon. Cereal with milk, toast with jam, bagels with cream cheese. Yogurt, fruit, waffles, oatmeal—and, of course, a big glass of orange juice. These are the foods that come to mind when most of us think of breakfast. They're America's breakfast foods, and there's nothing wrong with them.

But why are hash browns "breakfast" while a baked potato just . . . isn't? In some countries, breakfast just isn't breakfast without rice, or fish, or soup. America started as a British colony, but if you ever visit England, you might notice that somewhere along the way, our idea of a "traditional breakfast" diverged—few Americans are in the habit of starting the day with baked beans! The truth is, the foods we designate as "breakfast appropriate" are completely arbitrary. And there is no reason you *have to* eat "breakfast foods" for breakfast.

In Step 1, we agreed to set aside our assumptions about what constitutes a "good" breakfast. And so as you rethink the size of your breakfast, also consider what foods you choose, and give yourself permission to think outside the box when planning your morning menu. There's no reason you can't have a salad for breakfast, or a bowl of soup, or a cheese plate. Breakfast can be stir-fried veggies, a peanut butter sandwich, or anything else you want. Spend some time thinking about this. Are you crazy bored with the breakfast foods you eat? Or are you happy with them? If you think it might be fun to swap in some new foods, make a list of possibilities.

Put an egg on it! I often use last night's dinner as my breakfast inspiration. Throw a fried or poached egg on top of whatever veggie or grain you had the night before, and voilà! Breakfast. I've also been known to mix just about any leftover—veggies, salmon, even pieces of burger—into scrambled eggs or an omelet.

Step 3: Take the Breakfast Challenge

Some people know exactly what kind of breakfast suits them best. If that's you, then it's fine to skip the Breakfast Challenge. (Though you might want to give it a whirl just to be sure you know yourself as well as you think you do!) But some people don't have any clue whether they function best with a morning meal that's big, medium, small, or when they skip breakfast completely.

To pinpoint what size breakfast works best for you, you're going to conduct a study with just one subject—yourself. You'll do what the researchers do and make it scientific: Try four different breakfast strategies, and compare the results. You'll use these results to help you design your breakfast plan.

Directions for the Breakfast Challenge:

- Each day, eat the type of breakfast recommended for that day—no breakfast, small, medium, or large. For this challenge, use a range of about 20 to 35 grams of carbs and 250 to 500 calories, with your small breakfast falling at the low end of the range and your large breakfast falling at the high end.

- To keep things even, make each of your challenge breakfasts relatively high in protein and fat and relatively low in carbohydrates. (Remember, Target 100 limits carbs to 100 grams per day.) Eat similar foods each day, but adjust the *amounts* to hit the target carb or calorie count on the worksheet. For example, you may choose to eat a breakfast parfait made with yogurt, fresh berries, and granola, but the quantities of each will vary depending upon whether that day's breakfast is small, medium, or large.

- Using the Breakfast Challenge worksheet on the next page, check in with yourself throughout the day. For each check-in, take a few minutes to assess how you're feeling, both physically and mentally/emotionally. How is your energy level? How hungry do you feel? Are you experiencing food cravings or feeling satisfied? Are you eating more or less than usual for the rest of your meals and snacks? Are you experiencing any symptoms like headache, moodiness, or lethargy?

- After taking the four-day Breakfast Challenge, spend time reflecting on which breakfast size seemed to work best for you. Remember, you'll use your Breakfast Challenge results as a guideline to move forward—but you can always shift gears along the way.

- Keep in mind that your breakfast preferences may not be the same on weekends as they are on weekdays; you may want less or more because the rhythm of your day is different. You probably already have some idea of how weekends are different for you—maybe you always have a family breakfast on Saturdays, or you like to sleep in on Sundays and usually make do with coffee until lunch. Use that knowledge when you schedule your Breakfast Challenge, and try to include one or more weekend days.

THE BREAKFAST CHALLENGE

DAY 1 No Breakfast	DAY 2 Small Breakfast	DAY 3 Medium Breakfast	DAY 4 Large Breakfast
10 AM CHECK-IN			
LUNCHTIME CHECK-IN			
3 PM CHECK-IN			
DINNERTIME CHECK-IN			
8 PM CHECK-IN			
BEDTIME CHECK-IN			
OVERALL REFLECTIONS ON THIS DAY			

IS IT OK TO EAT THE SAME THING FOR BREAKFAST EVERY DAY?

In a perfect world, you'd eat a colorful variety of different super-nutritious breakfast foods. But the world isn't perfect, as we all know. If you find it easier to stick with one go-to breakfast most (or even all) days of the week, that's fine. Repeating one or two great breakfasts is far better than eating a wide variety of junk.

For some people—like my client Kit—having too many choices gets in the way of success. Kit struggled to figure out what to eat for breakfast each day, and this struggle often ended with her choosing poorly: grabbing a donut, bagel, or greasy breakfast sandwich at her local coffee shop on the way to work. I suggested she choose *one* healthy breakfast (she picked Greek yogurt, wild blueberries, and high-fiber granola) and eat it every day for a week. She gave it a try, and it worked like a charm, satisfying her hunger and removing her temptation to grab a donut or bagel. It was such a success that she decided to stick with it . . . permanently.

Eating the same breakfast every day was a huge relief for Kit because it removed the need for decision making, which for her was the hardest part of the process. At the grocery store, she'd buy a week's worth of Greek yogurt, granola, and frozen blueberries, which she'd measure out into a week's worth of containers. Instead of spending time and energy thinking about what to eat every morning, she just put it together and ate it—end of story. And throughout each day, she ate better knowing she'd already made one great, healthy choice in the morning.

This doesn't work for everyone—some people would lose their minds having the same breakfast every day. But if you think it would be an effective strategy for you, give it a try!

Step 4: Know Your Numbers

Once you've figured out what *size* breakfast suits you best, it's time to quantify your preferences. Using the words small, medium, and large is a good first step, but in order for you to be sure you're consistently eating the breakfast that best serves you and your weight-loss goals, we can move on to determining your ideal nutrient profile for this meal. (It should go without saying that, if you found during the Breakfast Challenge that you do best without breakfast, you can ignore this next section.) Remember, I want you to own your eating plan, so if you already have a plan you like, by all means, stick with it, and, over the course of this book tweak and adjust it so that it becomes more personalized and effective.

Either way, the following are some nutritional suggestions to keep in mind when planning your breakfasts.

Calories:

Let's start with calories, even though I am not going to talk about them much in this book. Wasting a lot of brain space on calories is unnecessary, and it makes weight loss far more complicated than it needs to be.

That said, as we work to uncover our perfect breakfast, we can use calorie *ranges* to hone our selections. For most people who choose to eat breakfast, a target of 250 to 500 calories works well, which is why I recommended it as the range for your

Breakfast Challenge. It allows for a filling, nutritious meal, while leaving a good amount of room for the remainder of the day's meals and snacks. You can use the results of your Breakfast Challenge to help you pinpoint quantities when you make your detailed plan in the next step—however, there is no need to keep track of calories in general.

Carbohydrates:

Focus on the Target 100 principle of eating only 100 grams of carbs per day. In practice, this means that whatever size morning meal you prefer, I recommend you limit your breakfast carbohydrates to 20–35 grams or fewer. This simple guideline will, like a domino effect, impact your entire meal.

Limiting carbs to 100 grams a day is the one and only food-related target in this book, and there is good reason for that. Studies suggest that a lower-carbohydrate diet is more likely to bring about weight loss. And what I know to be true, from years of experience, is that by creating awareness around this one number, you adjust the other macronutrient groups of fats and proteins by default. Protein and fats are much more satisfying and with this come less craving and less snacking. In order to limit your carbs, you will have to think about portion size, which will limit your caloric intake without requiring you to count a single calorie.

Additionally, watching carbs inevitably means cutting sugars—which is perhaps the single most important thing you can do for your health. Limiting yourself to fewer than 100 carbs a day will force you to look at labels and see where the hidden sugars lie. It will push you away from processed foods to whole foods that are naturally low in carbohydrates.

We'll talk much more about this in the next chapter, but for now, here are a few examples of common breakfast foods that fall on the lower and higher ends of the carbohydrate spectrum:

LOW CARB	HIGH CARB
Whole eggs	Cereal
Full-fat Greek yogurt	Bagels
Cheese	Flavored instant oatmeal
Canadian bacon	Flavored fat-free yogurt
Nut butters	Juices and smoothies
Low-carb tortillas	Frozen waffles

Protein:

Studies have also found that a higher protein diet is more likely than a lower protein diet to spur weight loss. Protein-rich foods are low in sugar and have staying power that helps keep cravings at bay. We'll go into more detail about protein later as well, but for now I suggest that you include at least one protein in your breakfast. Think eggs or Canadian bacon, salmon, steak, cheese, or sandwich meats. Even nuts and Greek yogurt pack a good amount of protein and will help get your day off to a satisfying start.

See the chart at right for some common breakfast foods that are great sources of protein.

PROTEIN FOOD LIST
Regular or turkey bacon
Eggs
Nuts/Nut butters
Greek yogurt
Cheese
Chicken sausage
Smoked salmon
Canadian bacon and ham
Soy milk
Beans

Healthy Fat:

Including fat in your breakfast helps chase away hunger throughout the morning by filling you up and keeping your blood sugar level stable. Choose foods like full-fat dairy, avocado, healthy oils, nuts, or fatty meats. In general, a good rule of thumb is to make sure that every breakfast has one serving of fat included. You may notice that there is a lot of overlap between the protein and fat categories—foods that do double duty like this are always a great choice!

See the chart at right for some fat options to consider.

HEALTHY FAT FOOD LIST
Bacon
Olive oil or butter
Eggs
Full-fat cheese or cream cheese
Avocado or guacamole
Full-fat yogurt
Nuts/Nut butters
Smoked salmon
Whole milk
Olives

Fruits and Vegetables:

In order to get ample amounts of vitamins, minerals, antioxidants, and all the nutrients that contribute to good health, I recommend including at least one serving of fruits or vegetables in your breakfast. This choice may use up a good chunk of the carbs allotted for this meal—just one cup of cantaloupe, for example, contains 14 grams of carbs—but the fiber in these foods can help keep you fuller longer.

I am a huge fan of trying to get a full serving or two of veggies in at breakfast. The recommendation is to get between five and nine servings of fruits and vegetables each day. I like to limit fruit to two or fewer of those servings, which leaves quite a few veggie servings to tackle. Knock a few out first thing in the morning in an omelet or even a smoothie!

Some of my favorite fruit choices include:

FRUIT	AMOUNT	CARBS (GRAMS)
Avocado	½ avocado	6
Clementine	1 clementine	9
Watermelon	1 cup	11
Strawberries	1 cup	12
Banana	½ medium banana	13
Raspberries	1 cup	14
Cantaloupe	1 cup	14
Apple	1 cup slices	15
Peaches	1 cup	15
Blueberries	1 cup	21

Some of my favorite vegetable choices include:

VEGETABLE	AMOUNT (RAW)	CARBS (GRAMS)
Spinach	1 cup	1
Mushrooms	1 cup	2
Celery	1 cup, chopped or sticks	3.5
Tomatoes	1 medium tomato	5
Bell peppers	1 cup, sliced	5
Asparagus	1 cup	5
Broccoli	1 cup	6
Onions	½ cup, chopped	8
Baby carrots	12 carrots	10
Potatoes	½ cup, diced	12

Step 5: Make a Plan

Now it's time to pull everything together and create your personalized one-week breakfast plan. As you've seen, breakfast is a simple meal that encompasses many decisions. Look back at the list on page 72, and take some time to consider what might need to change to accommodate your new plan. Remember, the changes you make to breakfast may not come easily at first. They will need to be triggered because they are not yet habit. What will you use to trigger your new behaviors in the morning? Could you set your alarm early, or leave yourself a sticky note as a reminder? Consider sitting down with a sheet of paper and using the Habit Change Key from Chapter One to plan your approach. There are also habit apps that "gamify" the formation of new habits, essentially acting as both trigger and reward—Google "habit app" to explore what's available.

Then, use the information you've gathered throughout this chapter—and the worksheet on the next pages—to create your own seven-day menu, with measured amounts of your favorite foods. (If you get stuck or overwhelmed, I've included a sample menu with a week's worth of delicious ideas after the worksheet.)

YOUR SEVEN-DAY BREAKFAST MENU

FOODS YOU'LL EAT, AND HOW MUCH	CALORIES (optional)	CARBS (grams)	PROTEIN? Y or N	FAT? Y or N	FRUIT/VEG? Y or N
MONDAY					
TUESDAY					
WEDNESDAY					
THURSDAY					
FRIDAY					
SATURDAY					
SUNDAY					

LIZ'S SEVEN-DAY BREAKFAST MENU

If it helps to have someone else provide ideas or a recommended breakfast menu, I'm happy to oblige! These breakfasts are medium to large in size—each is about 300 to 500 calories. Feel free to adjust amounts to fit the carb/calorie count that dovetails with the preferences you discovered during your Breakfast Challenge. And make sure to measure your ingredients—if you're pressed for time, get everything ready the night before.

MONDAY

Nutty Banana
½ banana (about 7 inches)
2 tablespoons nut butter spread on top

TUESDAY

Scramble in a Cup
2 eggs
¼ cup full-fat shredded cheddar cheese
Diced peppers
Diced onions
English muffin, toasted

Spray a microwave-safe mug with cooking spray. In the mug, combine eggs, cheese, peppers, and onions. Microwave on high for about 2 minutes. Flip perfect circle of eggs onto the English muffin.

WEDNESDAY

Yogurt-Berry Parfait
6 ounces plain or flavored 2 percent or full-fat Greek yogurt
1 cup fresh berries (raspberries, blueberries, blackberries, strawberries)
2 tablespoons slivered almonds or almond butter, to top

THURSDAY

Nutty Oatmeal Bowl
1 packet of plain oatmeal
1 tablespoon nut butter
1 cup raspberries

Prepare oatmeal and flavor with real vanilla, cinnamon, and/or stevia to taste. Mix oatmeal and nut butter; top with raspberries.

FRIDAY

Low-Carb Egg Wrap

2 eggs
2 pieces diced Canadian bacon
¼ cup shredded cheddar cheese
¼ cup spinach leaves
¼ cup salsa
Low-carb tortilla

Scramble eggs and heat Canadian bacon. Spoon eggs, Canadian bacon, cheese, spinach, and salsa into a low-carb tortilla.

SATURDAY

Easy Egg Cups

(Make on the weekend and save leftovers for quick, easy weekday breakfasts. For breakfast, enjoy two egg muffins with 1 cup of blueberries or similar.)

12 eggs
12 slices bacon
1½ cups shredded cheddar cheese
Salt and pepper to taste

Spray a muffin tin with cooking spray. Line each of the 12 muffin tins with 1 slice of bacon. Crack 1 egg into each muffin tin; sprinkle with cheddar. Bake at 350° for 25 minutes.

SUNDAY

Sunday Waffle Sundae

2 low-carb Eggo waffles
¼ cup whole-milk ricotta cheese
1 tablespoon sugar-free syrup
2 tablespoons chopped walnuts

Toast waffles. Top with ricotta cheese, syrup, and nuts.

YOU DID IT!

Congratulations, you've just taken a huge step toward creating new, healthier habits, and a personalized plan for lasting weight loss! The menu you've designed is just a beginning—in the next chapter, you'll generate more meal ideas as we explore the topic of food more fully. Most importantly, I want to empower you to see that no one knows you better than you do. Each of the targets in the following chapters is designed to get you moving in the direction of your healthiest self. As you progress, try to think of yourself as an ocean liner instead of a speedboat: allow for the fact that a ship turns slowly. Creating a new, healthier lifestyle is a big project. Let yourself focus on just one thing until you get it right. Then add another!

BREAKFAST ON THE RUN

It's great to have a leisurely breakfast, but let's face it, many of us are so rushed in the morning that grab and go is the only realistic option. Don't worry; you can still have a healthy, satisfying breakfast when you're short on time! Here are eight super-quick-prep breakfasts that will fit right into your plan—and your life:

- One small banana and a 100-calorie pack of almonds
- Two hard-boiled eggs and a piece of fruit
- A low-carb flour tortilla rolled up with ham and cheese
- Two egg muffins (see recipe on page 79)
- An English muffin with deli meat and cheese
- One Quest Bar and an apple
- One packet of Justin's all-natural almond butter on an apple
- A cheese stick and two hardboiled eggs

All of the above clock in around 300 calories, so adjust based on what size breakfast is best for you.

Chapter 4

FOOD THAT FUELS

Everyone told me this would be the first chapter you turned to. They warned me that you would ignore everything before and after "the food chapter" and dive in here, hoping to get started quickly. *I* am hoping that if this is true, you will reconsider—flip back, and start at the beginning. Otherwise, this will be no different from every other attempt you have made to lose weight. A single-minded obsession with food will not get you where you want to go. Let's get real. You likely already know what healthy eating looks like. This is probably not the first "weight loss" book you have purchased. If I told you we were going out to lunch together and there were just two choices on the menu, fettuccine Alfredo or grilled chicken with vegetables, would you know which one to order? Yup. *Food is not magic.* Don't get me wrong, food is a huge piece of the weight-loss equation, but our *behaviors* around food—whether we are preparing ahead of time, letting ourselves get too hungry, sitting down to eat without distractions— affect whether or not we are successful nearly as much as what foods we choose to eat. And our choices, more often than not, are affected by much more than knowledge of what we "should" eat. We are not robots! Stress, mood, sleep, and hydration all affect our ability to make healthy choices. Until you learn to see the bigger picture, and practice building new habits in a way that is personalized and sustainable, you won't create the lasting change you are looking for.

ONE SIMPLE TARGET

Aim for a limit of 100 grams of carbohydrates each day.

Target 100 has *one* target focused on food. *One* nutritional "rule" to follow. Just one. That means one number to remember and just one number to look up. I have logged hundreds of hours listening to what dieters want in a weight-loss program. They want fewer rules. They want something simple and livable. They want to be able to feel "normal" and eat at restaurants and with family and friends. I totally get this, because I want those very same things. What's more, I have seen, time and again, that simple is what *works*. So when I was developing this program, I looked for a guideline that would get results without introducing unnecessary complexity.

I first zeroed in on carbs after experimenting with an extremely low-carb diet as a guinea pig for one of my consulting gigs. After years of "low-calorie" and "low-fat" dieting, it was something of a shock. What perplexed me the most was the absence of hunger—I was insanely satisfied, because by lowering carbs I was basically forced into eating lots of protein (highly satisfying), fat (satisfying *and* decadent), and vegetables and fruits (filling and energizing). The specific diet I was on was super restrictive and I knew,

WHAT IS A CARB?

Our foods are made up of three macronutrients: carbohydrates, proteins, and fats. These are our three sources of dietary energy. Carbohydrates are the sugars, starches, and fibers found in fruits, grains, vegetables, and milk products. They are one of the basic food groups and are important to a healthy diet.

Carbohydrates are divided into two categories, simple and complex. *Complex carbs* are called "complex" because they require more work by your body to access the sugars they contain; they are higher in fiber and digest more slowly. *Unrefined complex carbs*—like fruits, vegetables, beans, and whole grains—have not been processed, and so they are the highest in fiber. This makes them more filling, which means they're a good option for weight loss. Because they are absorbed more slowly into your system, they help keep your blood sugar stable and control hunger. They also tend to be full of nutrients we need, like vitamins and minerals. Foods in this category also generally have fewer carb grams than foods that fall into other carb categories. *Refined complex carbs* are foods like white bread or fruit juice that have had most of the "processing" work your body would do during digestion already done for them: unfortunately, because they are stripped of their fiber and refined, they not only turn into sugar in your bloodstream more quickly than their unrefined counterparts, they also lose most of their nutritional value.

Simple carbs are basically sugars. Most of the simple carbs in our diet come in the form of sugars added to foods. You'll find them in white bread, cookies, candy, and also in places you wouldn't expect—like just about every packaged food, whether it is "sweet" or not. You probably know that eating complex carbs is better than simple carbs—unfortunately, nutrition labels don't tell you whether the carbohydrates are simple or complex. But don't worry: Because simple carbs have a very high number of carb grams in even a small amount, if added to food they will raise the carb count dramatically. By limiting carbs in general you will automatically limit simple carbs. Common simple carbs added to foods include:

- Sugar and brown sugar
- Corn syrup, high-fructose corn syrup, and corn syrup solids
- Glucose, fructose, and sucrose
- Fruit juice and fruit juice concentrates

based on my years of experience with my own dieting behavior and that of others, that it was in no way livable long term. How could I find a threshold of lower carbs that would create a sense of satiety and livability, while still leading to weight loss? Many carb-focused diets count "net carbs," allowing you to subtract fiber grams from your carbohydrate count because fiber has been shown to slow the absorption of carbs. The Atkins Diet, for instance, calls for fewer than 50 grams of "net carbs" per day. This is a pretty low limit, only really livable if you subtract enough fiber, and that seemed like a lot of work to me: looking up two numbers and doing subtraction, too? Math is not my strong point, and doing math when I am *hungry* is a nonstarter. I wanted one simple number that would work for everyone.

I started playing around with ratios and carb limits with my clients and found that a target of about 100 grams per day struck the ideal balance between livability and effectiveness. By limiting carbs to 100 grams, clients saw significant weight loss. Yet this threshold didn't mean they had to "give up" certain foods entirely. It was very doable, while still requiring what I consider the most important ingredient in any eating plan for weight loss: *awareness.* Clients had to start thinking a bit about the choices they made at each individual meal and how these would fit into their day as a whole. They had to begin to look at labels, and look up carb counts for foods that didn't have labels. Building and maintaining the habit of awareness around food is the one constant across the myriad successful weight-loss solutions I have helped to build or tried on my own as a "human guinea pig."

As with every target, the number 100 is what we *aim for*, not what we must hit every day to succeed. It is a guideline. "Close" counts. You didn't "miss" if your day comes in at 109 grams. What's more, though the target is a limit of 100 grams, there's no extra credit for keeping your carbs super low—this kind of mind-set will backfire; you won't feel as satisfied and will be more likely to quit. You can eat all 100 grams every single day and lose weight.

This is not a low-carb diet. The target of 100 grams of carbs will naturally move you away from processed foods and toward more nutritionally rich choices, but nothing is really "off limits." You can work in your favorite dessert or cocktail; it will simply serve to push out other carb-laden choices during your day.

WHY CARBS?

Why limit carbohydrates? Why not focus on calories, as so many other programs do? I am not the only person who will tell you that pretty much any diet will eventually result in some weight loss, if you stick to it. The problem is that "sticking to it" is hard—the stumbling block is always long-term livability, and how the plan fits into your real life once the motivation of the first few weeks has faded. My main goal was to make this as simple as possible, and the number of calories you should eat for weight loss depends on your height, weight, activity level, and metabolism. It is a moving target—it changes every time one of these other variables shifts. Limiting carbs to 100 grams will result in weight loss whether you are starting out at 300 pounds or 150, and there's no need to adjust the number as you lose weight or become more active. Many foods have few or negligible carbs and won't need to be counted at all, and because 100 is a relatively small number, as you become familiar with the carb contents of the foods you eat regularly, it will be easy (even for the math-challenged) to keep an eye on your carb goal without formal tracking.

What's more, cutting carbs has a domino effect on your nutritional choices that not only has a positive impact on your health, but will actually make "sticking to it" easier. Sugar is a carbohydrate, so the restriction to around 100 grams of carbs per day will keep your sugar intake—now known to be perhaps the most critical dietary factor for health—in check. Processed foods are filled with an addictive combination of sugars, fats, and chemicals that interfere with our hunger signals and undermine our willpower—but they also tend to be high in carbs, and so will be limited naturally by following this guideline. In addition, reducing the amount of room given to the macronutrient carbohydrate leaves an open space on your dietary plate. The options remaining to fill that space are the other two macronutrients—fats and proteins—or low-carb vegetables, all of which are naturally filling.

Fact-Free Foods

In my opinion, carbohydrates are where things have really gone wrong in our food supply in the last fifty years or so. The changes in the proteins we eat are nothing compared to the transformations in the realm of carbohydrates—we've created a staggering array of increasingly processed foods with the advance of food science and technology. The changes have happened so quickly that we had little time to evaluate whether this "progress" is good for us, and more and more current research is proving that we've had nutrition and weight loss pretty much all wrong.

Because I am so embedded in the nutrition and exercise world, I am often shocked to find my clients are holding on to diet "truths" that have long since been reversed. Eggs are not evil, our cholesterol level is not raised by cholesterol in our diet the way we once thought, and "low fat" doesn't mean "healthy." These are basics to me, but totally new concepts for many people I work with. They insist on egg-white omelets and love low-fat and nonfat products. They are back in the eighties in their understanding of what it means to eat well.

What we know now is that egg *yolks* contain more than 80 percent of the vitamins, minerals, and healthy fatty acids found in an egg. Sure, egg whites are full of protein, but without fat, you can't absorb it well! Egg yolks are also an excellent source of choline, which plays a role in burning fat. (Sometimes I feel really indignant, thinking about all those bland egg-white omelets I choked down years ago, trying to be "healthy.")

Just a few years ago, we really believed that fat was making us fat. Now we have come to understand that this is simply not true. Added sugars and refined carbs are the worst culprits—shunted directly to our fat stores, they raise blood-sugar levels and cause our bodies to become resistant to insulin, triggering an assortment of negative health effects. Many "low-fat" foods have had sugar added to them in lieu of fat. Full-fat dairy balances its sugars with fats and proteins that actually control how the sugars are released— without the fat, you lose that balance, and foods like skim milk and fat-free fruit yogurts are not the healthy options we've been taught they are. Yet I have to nearly shake clients to get them to eat full-fat dairy or whole eggs. They are terrified they'll gain weight because they have been taught that fat is the enemy, and giving up those old beliefs is difficult.

What's more, our food—especially in the realm of carbohydrates—has been increasingly modified in ways that most are unaware of. Modern wheat, for example, is nothing like the grain our grandmothers ate. After years of genetic manipulation aimed at making the grain grow faster, we have actually changed its biochemistry, and by the time it gets into a slice of bread it has been processed in a dozen different ways. As a result, we've seen a dramatic increase in wheat-related digestive problems—like celiac and IBS—and inflammation. In our effort to avoid fats, we created things like fake creamers and margarines that are full of synthetic ingredients, high-fructose corn syrup, and hydrogenated oils. These oils—you may know them as "trans fats"—lower your HDL (good) cholesterol, raise your triglyceride levels, and increase your risk of heart disease, and yet I have clients who still think margarine is better for them than butter! These oils are an example of a fat that truly is a killer—but it's one we created ourselves. We've seen an almost total reversal in what we know about food, weight loss, and health from the days of SnackWell's and diet soda. We were wrong, and now we are paying for it, with epic levels of obesity, diabetes, and metabolic syndrome.

The "diet industry" has been divided around simple debates such as fat versus sugar in part because there's money at stake. Identifying a new dietary scapegoat means identifying a new way to market food—during the low-fat craze, lots of foods that had *always* been fat free (like applesauce or plain popcorn) suddenly started putting it on their labels! Sometimes the scapegoat is something truly bad for you, as with trans fats, which have begun to be removed and will soon be a thing of the past. But it is important to be wary: The fact that something is labeled "no trans fats" doesn't mean it is good for you. Plenty of sugary, unhealthy foods are free of trans fats, and now the companies selling them have a new way to position their products as "healthful." The real reason we're all getting fatter isn't fat or even sugar on its own, as food marketers would have you believe. Instead it is the addictive combinations of fats, sugars, and salts alongside a rapidly changing environment of food availability and increasingly sedentary lifestyles.

So, what does this all mean? There will never be a shortage of newly emerging research and infighting among scientists and food companies about what we should and shouldn't eat. If we are honest, though, we all know what healthy eating looks like. **Eat foods that occur in nature, and limit processed and prepackaged foods as much as possible.** That is easier said than done in this environment, I know, but weight loss will be so much easier if you try. Processed foods are designed to make you want more. We *love* fat/sugar

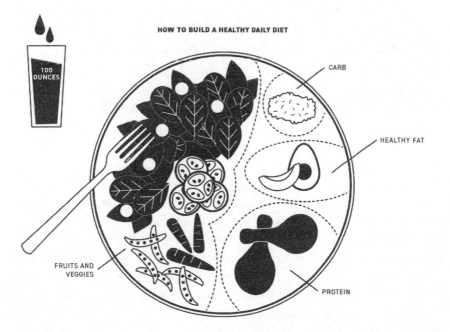

HOW TO BUILD A HEALTHY DAILY DIET

100 OUNCES

CARB

HEALTHY FAT

PROTEIN

FRUITS AND VEGGIES

combinations—candy bars, ice cream, French fries with ketchup. Brain scans and other tests reveal that eating these foods triggers the release of dopamine, a powerful neurotransmitter in the reward center of the brain; it's hard for *anyone* to resist eating too much of these. That said, any diet that tries to eliminate fat or sugar altogether will not only be incredibly hard to sustain, it will probably be bad for your health. Our brains run on glucose; without fat, many of the vitamins we need cannot be absorbed.

So instead we aim for balance. We begin to read labels before we buy. Most processed foods are high in carbohydrates—by limiting those, I am hoping to help you arrive at a mainly whole-foods–based diet.

The Research Supports Low-Carb Diets

It has become increasingly clear that diets low in carbohydrates are more effective than the standard low-fat diets long supposed to be the path to weight loss. Healthy fats are an important part of a healthy diet and fats really only become problematic when processed or paired with sugars and salts, both nutritionally and in terms of self-control. Plain butter is not something many people find themselves scarfing down in huge quantities; butter cookies, you can imagine, are another story! In fact, those put on a higher protein and fat regimen in one study saw significant improvement not only in weight loss and satiety (feeling satisfied), they even saw improvements in their cholesterol! One of the latest outcomes I found interesting was part of a yearlong study conducted by Tulane University. Researchers compared obese patients following a low-carb diet to those on a low-fat diet. The results were impressive: weight loss was three times higher in the low-carb group, with important upticks in lean mass (muscle) gained and in fat mass reduced:

LOW-FAT GROUP	LOW-CARB GROUP
• Average pounds lost: 3.9	• Average pounds lost: 11.7
• Fat mass lost: 0.3%	• Fat mass lost: 1.2%
• Lean mass lost: 0.4%	• Lean mass gained: 1.3%

The low-carb group also saw improvements in a variety of predictors of heart disease. This is a big deal, since a common concern about low-carb, high-fat diets has been their potential impact on heart health. Here, the low-carb group ended up with a higher HDL (good) to total cholesterol ratio than the low-fat group, which is a strong predictor of avoiding heart disease. They also had lower triglycerides and a lower calculated heart-disease risk score. Additionally, their LDL (bad cholesterol) dropped a bit more than that of patients in the low-fat group. To top it off, the low-carbers had a greater decrease in overall inflammation in the body—inflammation being linked more and more these days not just to heart disease but to many cancers.

The most important piece of this study, to me, was that when they looked at the food journals of those on the low-carb regimen, they found that though the diet they were supposed to be following called for only 40 grams of carbs per day—which is highly restrictive—patients were in fact averaging somewhere closer to 100 to 130 grams per day overall. While the researchers may have set out to look at the effects of an extremely low-carb diet, the benefits they found were all present on a diet that actually restricted carbs more moderately. These results also speak volumes to me about the importance of livability in any longer-term weight-loss attempt. Severe restriction was not sustainable even with the support of participating in a monitored study.

MAKING IT WORK

You've already transformed your breakfast. Now I'll walk you through some of the details of transforming the rest of your diet. As I've made pretty clear by now, I disagree with the approach of programs expecting you to do a complete 180 on day one, changing every aspect of your diet and your behaviors around food at once. Just the act of creating awareness around what you are eating is a giant behavior change to make. I often advise my clients to continue eating as they normally do for a day or two and just work on the habit of tracking carbs. This helps you see where the carbs live in your current diet and just how high your carbohydrate intake is to start with. Most clients come back to me exclaiming that they'd never realized how the foods they'd thought of as "healthy" are filled with sugars they never knew were there. A few of the biggest carb surprises are pasta sauces, "healthy" frozen meals, granola bars, flavored oatmeal, juices, and fruity yogurts. If you are eating hundreds upon hundreds of grams, perhaps it's best to begin by aiming to stay below 200 carbs for a week, then move to 150, and *then* zero in on 100. Remember, personalizing your plan makes it more likely that you will succeed.

Tracking (What About Portion Control?)

One of the great things about the target of 100 grams of carbs is that it won't require the obsessive tracking that calorie counting does, but, especially at the beginning, you *will* need to keep track of your daily carb count. You can do this in a very simple way in a small notebook or using the notes app on your phone. What's more, I always urge clients to actually write down what they are eating for a week or two at the beginning of any new shift in diet or routine. It creates a record that you can look to in the future while creating awareness of where change is needed in your day or even your week as a whole. I guarantee you will notice patterns that will surprise you and come in handy as you identify challenges and brainstorm solutions. Remember your habit loop—perhaps use alarms on your phone around the time of each meal to remind you to track, or begin preplanning and pretracking. As you become confident and begin to see where the carbs live in your diet and what foods are relatively free of them, don't even bother to track those like meats, eggs, cheeses, and so on that have negligible carb counts. Instead, simply record only the carb-heavy foods you eat throughout the day.

The bottom line is that you should *not* have to be tracking food your whole life! It is a difficult (and frankly tedious) habit to sustain, and it should be viewed as a tool to help you develop awareness, not as a substitute for that awareness. Eventually you won't need to formally track your carb grams at all, but it will remain a tool you can return to if your weight loss slows or you feel the need to reevaluate.

It won't take you long to see that the target of 100 grams of carbs per day is very doable, but will force some adjustments. For example, if you have oatmeal for breakfast—which is relatively high in carbs—you will likely need to cut down on the rice or pasta at dinner. But I'm not going to tell you what you must or must not eat, food by food. Every client says, "Just tell me what to eat," but I know that will never work. I don't know what you like, and the behavior modifications required for you to follow my prescribed meal plans would be far harder than what's necessary to lose weight. Alongside cultural and regional differences in food availability, personal preferences, levels of cooking expertise, and so on, we all have unique challenges. Some of us work at night, some have three kids, some have aging parents. You're going to have to dig in to your own lifestyle a little bit, and create your own meal plan based on *you* and our one simple target, using this foundation to find a way to eat the things you like while filling the majority of your day with healthy foods.

No Label? No Problem! Thanks to the internet and smartphones, practically every piece of information we could ever want is at our fingertips. To find the carbohydrate content of any food, you can simply search for the food itself. Just type "apple" into a search engine and its entire nutritional profile will come up right on the top of the page. There are also countless free apps—like Lose It!—you can use to find nutritional information, either by searching, scanning the food's bar code, or sometimes even taking a picture!

For clients who are used to detailed calorie tracking, my lack of emphasis on portions is hard to get used to. But of course, carb count directly relates to portion size. For example, there are just 22 grams of carbohydrate in a half cup of rice, while a full cup has close to 45. Beginning to think about portions in relation to the amount of carbohydrates in a food will be important.

PORTION SIZE GUIDE

BASIC GUIDELINES

| 1 CUP = BASEBALL |
| 1/2 CUP = LIGHT BULB |
| 1 OZ OR 2 TBSP = GOLF BALL |
| 1 TBSP = POKER CHIP |
| 3 OZ CHICKEN OR MEAT = DECK OF CARDS |
| 3 OZ FISH = CHECKBOOK |

GRAINS

| 1 CUP OF CEREAL FLAKES = BASEBALL |
| 1 PANCAKE = COMPACT DISC |
| 1/2 CUP COOKED RICE = LIGHT BULB |
| 1/2 CUP COOKED PASTA = LIGHT BULB |
| 1 SLICE BREAD = CASSETTE TAPE |
| 1 BAGEL = 6 OZ CAN OF TUNA |
| 3 CUPS POPCORN = 3 BASEBALLS |

DAIRY & CHEESE

| 1 1/2 OZ CHEESE = 3 STACKED DICE |
| 1 CUP YOGURT = BASEBALL |
| 1/2 CUP OF FROZEN YOGURT = LIGHT BULB |
| 1/2 CUP OF ICE CREAM = LIGHT BULB |

FATS & OILS

| 1 TBSP BUTTER OR SPREAD = POKER CHIP |
| 1 TBSP SALAD DRESSING = POKER CHIP |
| 1 TBSP MAYONNAISE = POKER CHIP |
| 1 TBSP OIL = POKER CHIP |

FRUITS & VEGETABLES

| 1 MEDIUM FRUIT = BASEBALL |
| 1/2 CUP GRAPES = ABOUT 16 GRAPES |
| 1 CUP STRAWBERRIES = ABOUT 12 BERRIES |
| 1 CUP OF SALAD GREENS = BASEBALL |
| 1 CUP CARROTS = ABOUT 12 BABY CARROTS |
| 1 CUP COOKED VEGETABLES = BASEBALL |
| 1 BAKED POTATO = COMPUTER MOUSE |

MEATS, FISH & NUTS

| 3 OZ LEAN MEAT = DECK OF CARDS |
| 3 OZ FISH = CHECKBOOK |
| 3 OZ TOFU = DECK OF CARDS |
| 2 TBSP PEANUT BUTTER = GOLF BALL |
| 2 TBSP HUMMUS = GOLF BALL |
| 1/4 CUP ALMONDS = 23 ALMONDS |
| 1/4 CUP PISTACHIOS = 24 PISTACHIOS |

MIXED DISHES

| 1 HAMBURGER (WITHOUT BUN) = DECK OF CARDS |
| 1 CUP FRIES = ABOUT 10 FRIES |
| 4 OZ NACHOS = ABOUT 7 CHIPS |
| 3 OZ MEATLOAF = DECK OF CARDS |
| 1 CUP CHILI = BASEBALL |
| 1 SUB SANDWICH = ABOUT 6 INCHES |
| 1 BURRITO = ABOUT 6 INCHES |

Especially in your first few weeks, I really do want you focusing only on carbs and staying true to portions there, as measured by grams. As I've said, this will force you into more satisfying foods. Your appetite will naturally decrease as you add proteins and fats, and you will naturally begin to eat less. But I am not saying this should become an all-you-can-eat buffet of proteins and fats. Here is some information to help you "eyeball" portions of various foods, if you feel like your awareness is lacking in this area:

Learn to listen to your body. Don't deprive yourself, but eat because you are hungry, *not* because "it's free." This is a huge problem I see when any food or group of foods is positioned as "unlimited." Target 100 does not limit portions beyond carbs (or even ask you to measure these foods) because they have a natural stopping point for most. If you find yourself overeating these low-carb foods—popping cheese into your mouth when you aren't hungry, eating past the point of fullness at mealtimes—take a step back and examine the habits, behaviors, or feelings surrounding that experience. I can almost guarantee that it has nothing to do with food. It doesn't take much of these more satisfying foods to dispel hunger and keep you full; overeating tends to be based in old patterns and emotions.

Low-Carb, No-Track Foods

These foods are so low in carbs that (except perhaps at the very beginning, as discussed above) there is no need to track them:

- Meats
- Fish
- Cheeses
- Oils and fats
- Eggs
- Nuts

Count-Less Vegetables

You don't have to count these guys either. These vegetables are low in carbs, full of water, filling, and nutritious. This is not a complete list—a good rule of thumb is that if a veggie has fewer than 6 or 7 grams of carbs in a cup, there's no need to count it (while we don't technically "subtract" fiber as part of the plan, a vegetable with six grams of carbs in a cup will have virtually no net carbohydrate effect). This makes tracking even easier: Had a big salad? Don't worry about the lettuce, but do track the dried cranberries you sprinkled on top!

- Asparagus
- Avocado
- Bok choy

- Broccoli
- Brussels sprouts
- Cabbage (or sauerkraut)
- Cauliflower
- Celery
- Cucumbers (or pickles without added sugars)
- Fennel
- Green beans and wax beans
- Greens (lettuce, spinach, kale, herbs, etc.)
- Mushrooms
- Jicama
- Peppers
- Radishes
- Sea vegetables (nori, seaweed)
- Snap peas
- Tomatoes
- Zucchini and summer squash

Count These, but Don't Count Them Out: Starchy Vegetables and Legumes

You may think they eat up too many of your carbs, but these are super foods. Defy the temptation to avoid these healthy staples. Lentils are a great source of protein, and many others in this category, like carrots and beets, are packed with vitamins. Potatoes and sweet potatoes can actually help keep blood sugar balanced, and including starchy vegetables will make it easier for you to cut down on things like bread without feeling deprived. Here you simply need to be aware of your portion size.

- Acorn and butternut squash *(16g carbs in 1 cup)*
- Beets *(13g carbs in 1 cup)*
- Carrots *(12g carbs in 1 cup)*
- Chickpeas/garbanzo beans *(40g carbs in 1 cup)*
- Lentils *(40g carbs in 1 cup)*
- Potatoes *(37g carbs in 1 medium)*
- Spaghetti squash *(8g carbs in 1 cup)* (Makes a great pasta alternative!)
- Sweet potatoes *(26g carbs in 1 small)*

A Word About Fruit

The emerging research shows that one of the most dangerous sugars, in terms of impact on weight gain and overall wellness, is fructose. Fructose is the sugar that occurs in fruits, and it is also added to many processed foods as a sweetener. We now know that up to one-third of the fructose we consume gets immediately sent into fat storage. Because it is so high in sugar and the kind of sugar it contains is uniquely likely to interfere with weight loss, I suggest you limit fruit to two servings a day while you are trying to lose weight. We as a species are not particularly used to having an unlimited supply of every fruit, year round, and our bodies haven't evolved to handle this level of fruit (or sugar) consumption. Today, bananas, mangoes, and clementines are at our fingertips all day, every day, but not so long ago there were lengthy stretches where our only exposure to fruit might be through jam or other canned goods. Before long-distance air and refrigerated truck transport became relatively cheap and commonplace, we simply didn't have fruit in winter months. Fruits are full of vitamins, and many (especially berries) are nutritional powerhouses—they should absolutely be included in your diet! By limiting yourself to two or fewer servings a day, however, you will see greater success.

Protein and Staying Satisfied

One of the benefits of lower carb intake is that it often leads, indirectly, to an increase in intake of protein. Fewer carbs plus more protein is a solid recipe for fat loss. Believe it or not, getting more protein into your diet can help you lose weight even in the absence of other significant dietary changes. I explain it to clients this way: Protein is very difficult for your body to break down. For this reason, it keeps you fuller longer—your body even burns extra calories just processing it and moving it through your system. Carbs are like kindling for your metabolism; you burn through them fast. Protein and fats burn slowly and steadily.

You cannot hope to reduce your carb intake—or stick to any weight-loss plan—without sufficient protein. You will be a hangry mess. You know the quote "man shall not live on bread alone"? Well, guess what: You can't live on salad alone, either. Look to add some protein to each meal. More protein will give your meals more staying power and keep your blood sugar on an even keel—and keep you from reaching for carbs midmorning or midafternoon.

Good Sources of Protein

There are lots of ways to add protein to your diet, even if you don't eat meat. Here are some of my favorites:

FOOD (GRAMS OF PROTEIN)
Chicken or turkey, 3 ounces (27)
Lean beef, 3 ounces (23)
Salmon, trout, fresh tuna, halibut, 3 ounces (23)
Tilapia, 3 ounces (21)
Canned tuna, 3 ounces (20)
Shrimp (20)
Plain Greek yogurt, 6 ounces (17)
Cottage cheese, ½ cup (14)
Milk, 1 cup (8)
Pasta, 1 cup cooked (8)
Beans, ½ cup cooked (8)
Cheese, 1 ounce (medium hard—cheddar, Swiss, etc.) (7)
Nuts, 1 ounce (7)
Egg, 1 large (6)
Oatmeal, 1 cup cooked (6)

Don't Fear Fat

Fat, too, is an important part of a healthy diet—not "*even*" if you are trying to lose weight, *especially* if you are trying to lose weight. I've said this several times already, but it is so important to get over your fear of fat. Here's why:

- Pairing a carb with a fat helps slow the absorption and keep your blood sugar stable.
- Fats help you stay satisfied and fight cravings.
- Certain fats, like those found in fish, nuts, and avocados, contain omega-3 and omega-6 fatty acids, which have been shown to fight inflammation and have a host of health benefits.
- Many vitamins and nutrients cannot be absorbed by the body without fat.

It is vital that you include things like fuller-fat dairy, nuts, fish, and healthy oils in your diet. Drizzle olive oil over a salad of fresh tomatoes, mozzarella, and basil. A splash of cream (which, by the way, has almost no carbs) in your coffee can feel luxurious, and radishes with butter and salt make a healthy, pleasantly French-seeming snack. I promise, it won't kill you.

The Importance of Indulgence

I love rolling this plan out to my clients. It is so simple—only one target to aim for—that they grab on to it immediately, feeling confident and committed. But while it is simple, it is not always easy. I am asking you to grasp a concept that requires some maturity: flexible restraint. "Flexible restraint" refers to a diet methodology of putting a *moderate* level of control on eating to achieve weight-loss success. Those who learn to "dabble" with indulging, who learn to eat pizza, drink wine, and even have some chocolate in moderation, are practicing "flexible restraint." Eating habits that incorporate flexible restraint have enough structure to place some limits on the kinds or amounts of food you consume, while also avoiding the resentment that comes with feeling deprived or restricted. The target of 100 carbs a day will allow you to incorporate some of the "high-carb" foods and drinks you love into your life. It will allow for small indulgences. And because 100 is a target, not a check box, a day that misses the mark is just a day, not a disqualification. I wholeheartedly encourage you to take advantage of this flexibility, to learn to indulge in controlled ways. This entire book is about changing your mind-set, moving from extreme, narrow ways of thinking to a more holistic understanding of wellness and weight loss. In the past, you may have told yourself that an indulgence meant that you had "messed up" and were "off plan." Instead, I am asking you to actually plan indulgences, and create habits that contain them—like sharing a dessert or buying a single-serving bag of chips. If you are miserable, you will inevitably fall off *whatever* plan you are following and zigzag right back to your old habits. In a study of dieters, participants saw much greater success if they learned the habit of flexible restraint alongside modifying unrealistic expectations of weight loss. Those who are successful adopt a style of livable, enjoyable, healthier eating long term.

When you learn to indulge:

1. **Food loses its control over you.** Figuring out how to handle indulging means you have strategies and routines in place to account for unexpected eating situations or to recover quickly from stumbles. When you allow for indulgence, you also realize this is not the "last time" you will ever be able to eat a certain food. Knowing a food is forbidden makes us immediately crave it. Knowing you can incorporate it—regularly if you want—in a moderate way removes the heightened emotions.

2. **You learn to trust yourself.** At first, you might be afraid to indulge. Maybe you don't believe you can handle the flexibility and feel safer sticking to only a few foods you know—or those you know you can control yourself around. That might work for a while, but you can't live that way indefinitely. Things come up. Change happens. It's smart to add some new strategies and routines aimed at allowing and planning for

indulgence rather than relying on pure willpower. When you learn to indulge, you trust that you can have dinner out with friends and still remain in control.

3. **You lose more weight—because you're happier.** If you can go out to dinner with friends, enjoy some of your favorite foods, and even have a glass of wine, all without "ruining your diet," you'll be more content, and more likely to stick with your healthy lifestyle. It's not rocket science: When you are happy, you feel more confident and motivated. Those good feelings can help you lose weight.

The Truth About Alcohol and Weight Loss

I wanted to make sure to address this because I am a real wino. I lost sixty-five pounds and continued to enjoy alcohol as I lost the weight, but I certainly wish someone had given me the inside scoop on alcohol and weight loss earlier. It probably slowed my progress more than any other single habit. Don't worry, I'm not gearing up to tell you to toss the rosé, but with alcohol, calories and carbs don't tell the whole story, and it is something you should be aware of.

First, let's talk about the physiology. Alcohol is a toxin (which is why we say we are "intoxicated" when we drink). Our bodies want to rid themselves of toxins as fast as they can, so when we consume alcohol it is immediately converted to a quick energy source called *acetate*. Acetate can't be stored, so it must all be burned off before our bodies return to burning carbs or fats or proteins. So imagine that the carbs and fats you've consumed that need to be burned for weight loss have just been sent to the end of the line. They may end up stored as fat if the body has enough quick fuel from the alcohol/acetate. You can think about drinking as pushing the pause button on your metabolism.

Compounding this problem is that alcohol has more calories per gram than either carbs or proteins, clocking in at 7 per gram. One of my suggestions that really gets people's attention is to imagine you are actually

Don't you dare give up what you love. I have never seen anyone be successful with weight loss without finding a place for the things that make their life worth living. For me, it's wine and chocolate. For Jennifer Hudson, it was sushi and chicken wings.

having a tiny hot fudge sundae for each drink you consume. I say that because the numbers, on paper, can look relatively harmless, but the reality is more complicated than numbers show. Here are a few reasons why:

- **Dehydration.** As your body tries to rid itself of the toxins in alcohol, it sheds both water and vital minerals like potassium, magnesium, and sodium, leaving you dehydrated. Dehydration is often mistaken for hunger the next day. It also makes it harder for the body to access stored energy in the form of glycogen, and that, along with the loss of minerals, drives us to sweet or salty foods—usually high in carbs.
- **Loss of inhibition.** I know from personal experience that after more than one drink, it's harder to stick to my plans for healthy eating. Several studies point to the fact that alcohol can increase appetite in the short term, and combined with lowered impulse control, the result is often late-night foraging for snacks.
- **Lack of good sleep.** You may have noticed that drinking allows you to fall asleep quickly and deeply . . . and then you find yourself wide awake in the middle of the night. This is because alcohol disrupts REM sleep, our most restorative rest of the night. Lack of REM sleep has been linked to excess production of cortisol and other hormones that disrupt metabolism. Additionally, waking exhausted can lead to feelings of hunger as your body searches for fuel, avoidance of exercise due to lack of energy, and impaired focus and motivation.
- **Sugar cravings.** Alcohol causes an increase in insulin secretion, which leads to low blood sugar, which leads to cravings. After a night of drinking or even during, you may find yourself reaching for high-carb treats. Carb cravings are a biological response to low blood sugar and are often stronger than your willpower—they're designed to be.

All this said, I am not one who believes you have to give up drinking altogether in order to lose weight. We've all seen the studies that show wine, in particular, can be practically a health tonic, and as I've said, I'm a big proponent of small indulgences. As long as you are aware of the challenges posed by alcohol that aren't reflected by the carb count, there is no reason you can't continue to enjoy a drink or two. I have arrived at my own set of guidelines that allow me to lose weight without losing the wine:

1. **Moderation is truly the key—along with self-knowledge.** Be honest with yourself about the amount you are consuming and the effect it has on your eating and exercise. Personally, I can't drink more than once a week

if I want to lose weight, and I can't have more than three drinks. Figure out your own equation. Maybe you can have a single glass of wine with dinner. Maybe a single glass of wine makes you feel deprived, and you'd rather have two, but less often. Maybe you find when you drink at home you snack too much, so you decide to only drink when you're out.

2. **Eat with your drinks!** Look for a protein and fat combo to level blood sugar and help stave off hunger and cravings. Think salami and cheese or hummus and carrots.

3. **Have a glass of water in between every drink.** This will help you avoid dehydration, slow you down, and ensure you don't gulp your drink because you're actually thirsty.

4. **Use others to keep you accountable.** I often rely on my husband or a close friend to remind me to drink water and stop after a certain number of drinks. On nights when I can't afford to drink, I volunteer to be the designated driver. It makes abstaining easy because I would never go back on my promise to get everyone home safely.

Plan for Success

Use what you learned in the last chapter as you transformed your breakfast! Take the time to sit down with some scratch paper and think through your schedule, your preferences, your challenges (Do you shuttle the kids to baseball on Tuesdays? Have a lunch meeting every other Monday?), and do a little research into the carb content of your favorite meals and go-to snacks. You can find the nutrition information for hundreds of recipes on the internet. Go ahead and think up new things you might want to try, and be creative, but also be realistic about how much energy you have after work or how much time in the morning—don't expect yourself to change what you eat *and* transform from someone who relies on convenience foods into a gourmet chef. Get into the habit of meal planning for the week ahead, if you aren't already. Remember, planning ahead means more than deciding what you will eat, it also means making sure you have the ingredients you need and blocking off time in your schedule for preparing food *and* for the planning and prep steps as well.

Below, you'll find three glimpses of what a day of eating might look like on Target 100. After that is one of my favorite worksheets: the "5-5-5 Worksheet." Use it to record five breakfasts, five lunches, and five dinners that you know you'll like and will keep you within your carb goals (there is also a place to list snacks). Record the carb counts alongside your meal and snack ideas, and then use the worksheet as a meal-planning shortcut when you need it.

THREE DIFFERENT DAYS ON TARGET

DAY ONE: JEN

Jen likes to start with a big breakfast and taper her meals down during the day, ending with a small dinner and nothing to eat after. Her main indulgence each day is a serving of dark chocolate in the afternoon.

BREAKFAST

Omelet

2 eggs 1g
Spinach 0g
¼ cup shredded cheddar cheese 1g
Mushrooms 0g
¼ cup diced tomatoes 2g
2 slices Canadian bacon 2g
Coffee with 2 tablespoons half and half 1g

→ **7G CARBS**

LUNCH

Open-faced tuna sandwich

Tuna 0g
2 tablespoons full-fat mayo 0g
English muffin, whole grain 22g
Sliced red pepper and onion 0g

→ **22G CARBS**

TREAT

½ bar dark chocolate (70% or higher) 15g
. . . . (depending on brand)

→ **15G CARBS**

SNACK

1 7-ounce container Greek yogurt, plain, full fat . . 8g
1 cup raspberries 15g

→ **23G CARBS**

DINNER

Grilled chicken with mustard glaze

4 ounces chicken breast 0g
2 teaspoons Dijon mustard 0g
Tarragon 0g
2 teaspoons lemon juice 0g
Olive oil 0g
Sweet potato with butter 27g
1 cup spinach cooked with garlic and olive oil 0g

→ **27G CARBS**

TOTAL FOR THE DAY: **94G CARBS**

DAY TWO: ABBY

Abby is a vegetarian. She prefers smaller, snack-like meals throughout the day.

BREAKFAST

Oatmeal, 1 cup, cooked 27g
topped with 2 tablespoons SunButter . . . . 5g   → **32G CARBS**
Coffee, black. 0g

SNACK #1

Baby carrots (about 10). 10g
¼ cup hummus. . . . . 9g   → **19G CARBS**

SNACK #2

2 ounces white cheddar cheese. 1g
Almonds (single-serving pack) . . . . 4g   → **5G CARBS**

SNACK #3

Apple, small, sliced. 21g
2 tablespoons almond butter . . . . 3g   → **30G CARBS**

SNACK #4/DINNER

Deconstructed veggie burger
   Veggie burger, sliced 10g
               (depending on brand)
   ½ avocado, sliced 6g
   ½ medium tomato, sliced . . . . .5g   → **22G CARBS**
   1½ ounces blue cheese crumbles 1g
   Drizzle olive oil, salt, pepper .0g

TREAT

5 ounces wine . . . . 5g   ⟶ **5G CARBS**

TOTAL FOR THE DAY: **107G CARBS**

DAY THREE: MORGAN

Morgan prefers a small breakfast. She is on the run most of the day but enjoys cooking dinners, saving most of her carbs for the evening.

BREAKFAST

Everything Bagel Thin 25g
1 ounce goat cheese. . . . . 0g → **28G CARBS**
¼ avocado, smashed, with sea salt. 3g

LUNCH

Salmon salad
    4 ounces salmon. 0g
    Salad of "no count" greens and veggies. . . . . .0g → **1G CARBS**
    Olive oil and balsamic vinegar dressing 1g

SNACK

Peanut butter Power Crunch bar . . . . 10g ⟶ **10G CARBS**

DINNER

Soy Ginger Salmon and Sweet Potatoes,
homemade from recipe on page 236 . . . . 30g → **30G CARBS**

TREAT

½ cup Häagen-Dazs vanilla ice cream 21g
½ cup strawberries, sliced . . . . 7 → **28G CARBS**

TOTAL FOR THE DAY: **97G CARBS**

5-5-5 WORKSHEET

BREAKFASTS:

1. _____
2. _____
3. _____
4. _____
5. _____

LUNCHES:

1. _____
2. _____
3. _____
4. _____
5. _____

DINNERS:

1. _____
2. _____
3. _____
4. _____
5. _____

SNACKS:

1. _____
2. _____
3. _____

THE PROBLEM WITH PERFECTION

When clients start this plan and have trouble, I inevitably find they are imposing restrictions that weren't there, shooting for as low a carb value

The definition of the word "diet" is "the kinds of food that a person, animal, or community habitually eats." What if you stopped thinking of your diet as a restrictive, prescriptive regimen and instead as just the particular assortment of foods you habitually eat? Changing your perspective on that one word can change your whole attitude.

as possible and just generally trying to be weight-loss overachievers. If this sounds like you, let me say: This will doom you to failure. For one thing, you need carbs—they aren't your enemy! For another, the cycle of diet extremism leads nowhere. The motivation behind this book was my desire to give you the guidelines and tools to create lasting change. I could have written a plan to get you to drop as much weight as humanly possible in two or four or six weeks, but I didn't, because what's the point? I know, I absolutely know that in six months you'd probably be back where you started. Each and every time I, or one of my clients, has tried to scale the wall of weight loss in a single jump we've ended up flat on our backs.

I get the chance to meet and work with hundreds of people each year. Most are totally confused in their understanding of what is "healthy" and believe that to make any progress, they will have to jump from where they are straight into a diet of foods like spelt and almond milk. I got to the place where I was sixty-five pounds heavier by checking out, believing that I might as well do nothing because what I'd need to do to lose all that weight was going to be awful and extreme. In truth, I have seen that small changes and transitioning to healthier food choices over time are the fabric of real results—without frustration, deprivation, or alienating you from your social life. What works is understanding what goes into making these changes, giving ourselves credit for our efforts, and checking in to make sure the changes we are making are right for us. I am still learning and making adjustments as my life evolves and my children grow, as I experiment and discover how certain foods make me feel. This is not a static process—what is right for you today may not be ten years from now.

Super-restrictive diet plans ignore the most important variable of all: you. For example, many eliminate whole food groups, like dairy. Some people find removing dairy makes them feel great; I personally have no issues with dairy, and eliminating it makes me feel totally deprived and cranky. You should never be afraid to say, "That doesn't work for me." Last year, we decided to try getting a share of vegetables delivered to us weekly from a local farm. Friends of ours were huge fans of this, and we had heard it was fun and that the vegetables were delicious. Well, the vegetables *were* delicious . . . but they also ended up feeling like a full-time job. Each week I found myself with a giant box of veggies that I had not chosen, and sometimes had no idea how to prepare. Then it was a weeklong race to try to use everything up before the next box. In the end, lots of produce went bad, it was expensive, and I decided that it was not for us. But I am still glad I tried it! Every experience teaches us something and moves us closer to understanding ourselves. I always tell my clients to think of trying new wellness habits like trying on new shoes. If the shoes don't fit, you don't feel like a "failure," or force yourself to keep walking around in them, limping and miserable—you try another pair! Remove the weight of expectation from your shoulders, and stop expecting instant perfection.

NOW FORGET EVERYTHING I SAID

On that note, I am really going to blow your mind. This is *my* system. I came up with it after years in the weight-loss industry in an honest attempt to offer you something that would be effective, simple, and hopefully even teach you a little something about nutrition. But, guess what? I don't mind if you use another system, or take parts of mine and meld them with other things that have worked for you in the past. Why? Because that is where real success lies. Not in blindly following the dictates of others, but in finding what works for you and will continue to work long term. I have coached thousands of people, and no two of them are doing exactly the same thing when it comes to food. Food holds tremendous meaning for most of us. It is embedded in our family and cultural traditions, our social rituals, our memories. How could there be a one-size-fits-all solution?

HABIT LIBRARY

1. Schedule a specific time for weekly meal planning and to stock up on anything you need.
2. Add a fruit or vegetable to each meal.
3. Take ten or fifteen minutes as you unload groceries to chop and prep raw veggies for snacks.
4. Pre-measure individual portions of snacks into plastic bags.
5. Create a recipe book filled with family favorites to glance at when inspiration is low.
6. Make a "staples" shopping list in your phone or to keep in your purse at all times.
7. Start carrying healthy snacks with you in your bag or purse.
8. Start bringing lunch to work.
9. Make a list of three healthy delivery options in your neighborhood and keep the list in plain sight, for instance on your fridge.
10. Look up restaurant menus ahead of time to identify low-carb options and decide what you will order.
11. Designate a day of the week to eat vegetarian, à la "Meatless Monday."
12. Drink a full glass of water before you begin eating your meal.
13. Add a fruit or vegetable to every snack.
14. Sign up for a healthy recipe newsletter.
15. Try a meal-kit delivery service like Blue Apron or Plated.
16. Try grocery delivery to avoid the temptation of the grocery store.
17. Try measuring portions at dinnertime for one week. Leave a food scale or measuring utensils and cups out where you can see them.
18. Order an appetizer as your main meal when dining out.
19. Start each dinner this week with a green salad.
20. Try a new-to-you fruit or vegetable.
21. Try doubling a healthy recipe and using the leftovers for the next day or two.
22. Try cooking a new healthy grain—think bulgur, quinoa, or farro.
23. Brush your teeth after every meal to send a clear signal to your brain that you are done eating.
24. Spend a week alcohol free.
25. For one week, track how you feel before and after meals to gauge satiety and learn more about your hunger signals.

Chapter 5

WATER, WATER, EVERYWHERE

I 'll bet you are tired of hearing that you should drink more water. It is mentioned in almost every weight-loss plan or article about staying healthy. Still, it is often treated as a footnote or an aside, something we all know we should be doing but that is simply icing on the cake—definitely not as important as your food plan or exercise regime. By now you know that the weight-loss process is complex and cannot be reduced to a singular focus on any one variable. It is an equation affected by your environment, history, emotional responses, social pressures, and most importantly, your habits. All that said, there is a reason I am devoting a whole chapter to what many would give only a page: nothing has affected more of the people I've worked with, more dramatically, than hydration.

"Seriously?" I can hear you saying. Yup. The truth is, when it comes to weight loss, the importance of water is hard to overstate. And I often tell my clients, should they let their healthy choices fall by the wayside for a while and feel overwhelmed about how to get started again, to ease into their return by focusing just on water intake. Much like asking you to focus only on breakfast, it is simple, doable, and the effect is magical—it snowballs into other changes in ways you might find surprising.

A CASCADE OF EFFECTS

Your body depends on water to survive. Every cell, tissue, and organ in your body needs water in order to work correctly. You've probably heard that up to 60 percent of your body is composed of water, but let's get more specific: The brain and heart (arguably the two most important weight-loss organs) are 73 percent water, and the lungs about 83 percent. The skin is 64 percent water; the muscles and kidneys, 79 percent. Even our bones are 31 percent water! Stomach health, skin health, kidney and urinary tract

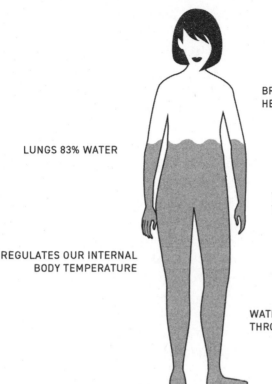

BRAIN AND
HEART 73% WATER

LUNGS 83% WATER

WATER FLUSHES TOXINS FROM
THE BODY VIA URINE AND SWEAT

REGULATES OUR INTERNAL
BODY TEMPERATURE

WATER CARRIES OXYGEN TO CELLS
THROUGHOUT THE BODY

health, and even cholesterol regulation are all affected by hydration or the lack thereof.

Hydration also plays a key role in helping your body maintain its temperature, remove waste, and lubricate joints. Keeping your body hydrated helps your heart pump blood through the vessels more easily, meaning your heart doesn't have to work as hard.

Let's talk about the symptoms of dehydration. Most likely you have felt them, but—as the majority of people do—incorrectly attributed them to hunger. An important part of Target 100 is getting to know your body, learning to distinguish hunger from thirst, emotional hunger from real hunger, and the need for sleep from the need for food. Dehydration symptoms include actually feeling thirsty or having a dry mouth, but also headaches, constipation, and dizzy spells. Another symptom of dehydration I often experience is impaired memory and loss of concentration. Dehydration can make you feel foggy and fatigued, affect your mood, and even give you muscle cramps.

If you aren't sure whether you're dehydrated, the color of your urine is a pretty good indicator. If it is clear or a light-straw color, then you are properly hydrated. If it is darker, guess what? You are dehydrated. Incredibly, it is estimated that 75 percent of the American population is chronically dehydrated. That is a staggering number. That means that, as you read this, *you* are probably dehydrated. (If I were you, I would get up and have a glass of water right now!)

A word about the spate of fad detox diets that have swept through our culture: These diets are based on the idea that we need to "detox" our bodies from whatever substances in food or the environment that the diet has deemed toxic. Often these programs advocate extreme regimens (like subsisting only on juice) with little basis in science or medicine. The simple fact is that your body is already equipped with a powerful detoxification apparatus—from amazing organs like your liver and kidneys to your respiratory and lymph systems. This apparatus works extremely well—*as long as it is hydrated enough to do the job it was built to do*. Many cleanses and detox protocols include extreme hydration to flush out toxins. How about if we simply hydrate and flush on a daily basis?

Hydration is a serious piece of your overall health and wellness. It is not an optional extra or something to do twice a year as part of a short-lived "cleanse." We must build the habit and make it a part of our daily lives.

WATER AND WEIGHT

If you aren't drinking enough water, your weight loss will be slow and seem endlessly difficult. If you are chronically dehydrated (and remember, you probably are), the parts of your body that depend on water to function are running on fumes. Just like a car low on oil, systems begin to grind to a halt. When there isn't enough water, your body does what it must to keep you alive—it slows everything down. Everything! Your body is a machine designed for survival, and it could not care less about your weight-loss goals. It has a responsibility to keep your heart pumping and your cells dividing and your eyes tearing. And so to conserve water, it will slash your metabolism. The carbohydrates and proteins our bodies use for energy are metabolized and transported by water in the bloodstream. Low on water? Your body orders that transportation brought to a screeching halt. Save every nutrient, it instructs, because something is obviously wrong. Can you imagine? Just by being dehydrated you are personally slowing down your own metabolism.

Dehydration will continually drive you to seek food when you are not hungry. I will say this several times in this book: *Your body is smarter than you*. If you are not giving it the water that it needs, it will drive you to eat, hoping to extract water from the food you take in. This strategy was very valuable when the majority of foods that people consumed were fruits and vegetables, filled with water and nutrients. It worked to keep people without adequate water supply alive. In our modern environment, triggering hunger in a body stressed by dehydration is unlikely to make us reach for a juicy apple—for one thing, dehydration makes us crave salt as our body tries to balance our electrolytes, and salty snacks are readily available. Instead, we reach for anything sweet or salty, and today this likely comes in a package, and is completely lacking the water we need, despite the fact that this is what sent us looking for a snack in the first place.

Trying to lose weight while dehydrated is physically and emotionally exhausting. You will be plagued by cravings and frustrated by feeling that you must exert heroic amounts of willpower for little progress. On the other hand, a University of Washington study found that one glass of water stopped hunger pangs for nearly 100 percent of participants. Can you imagine avoiding all that drama with just a glass of water?

WHY SO HIGH?

Target 100 asks you to aim for 100 ounces of water a day. You may be wondering why I am asking you to set a target of 100 ounces when the most commonly recommended daily intake is eight glasses of water a day—about sixty-four ounces. There are two reasons.

First, over my many years of experience I have consistently observed that when the goal is sixty-four ounces, my clients fall short. They get to around fifty and subconsciously feel that they're "close enough." And while many agencies use the recommendation of eight glasses a day/sixty-four ounces, the National Academy of Medicine determined the ideal water intake— enough to fully replenish the body without overwhelming the cells—is actually approximately sixteen eight-ounce cups (128 ounces) for men and eleven eight-ounce cups (eighty-eight ounces) for women. Depending on your weight and whether you engage in strenuous exercise, you may need even more. And guess what? You can't really have too much water in a day. Dangerous intakes of water don't occur until you are ingesting gallons upon gallons in a relatively short period of time. In a healthy body, extra water in your system is simply flushed out as waste. My goal in setting a target of 100 ounces is to get each of you to *at least* sixty-four ounces—and hopefully far beyond. Raising the target means you will have to work harder and more consciously to accomplish the goal.

Why does an eight-ounce glass of water look so *big* when even an eight-ounce glass of wine is never a struggle to power through? Try drinking your water out of a wine glass and watch your perspective change!

Secondly, Target 100 was designed to be the absolute easiest weight-loss program I could create. In order to find out how much water you should be drinking, many diets and health programs ask you to perform some sort of calculation based on body weight, and then add a certain number of ounces for each however-many minutes of exercise you perform and so on. Remember, I *am* you. I have read those books. I have looked at that equation and thought "no thank you" and simply didn't bother to do it. And even when I did? I couldn't remember the number, because it changed every time I lost a pound or switched up my exercise routine! Redoing my water "calculation" every week? Sorry, not gonna happen. As with every needlessly complicated plan, I inevitably ended up feeling disinterested, defeated, frustrated, or confused. I don't want you confused. I don't want you struggling to remember numbers and calculations, or worrying about updating everything as soon as you make progress. Think "100" for every target and you are all good, I promise. Even if you are starting at a higher weight or are an avid cycler and your "actual" ideal water intake is more like 110 ounces, 100 ounces will be *great*—and almost certainly better than whatever you are getting now.

Do You Need a Sports Drink? Sports drinks provide carbohydrates for energy plus minerals to replace electrolytes (sodium, potassium, magnesium) lost in your sweat. They are designed to rapidly replace fluids and to increase the sugar (glucose) circulating in your blood. But they are rarely necessary for the majority of people using them. The marketing around these drinks, however, has been very effective. Many of my clients believe they "need" to replace electrolytes after just about any amount of exercise. Unless your activity was strenuous and lasted an hour or more, put down the Gatorade. Even then, be wary, and take a moment to look at the nutrition label. Most have nearly as much sugar and carbs, if not more, than soda. Water and a post-exercise snack will serve you far better.

So the goal is 100 ounces per day—and I don't count just anything against those ounces. No, I am asking you to take in 100 ounces of *water*. Why? Because it is what your body wants. Also, if there are any bad habits hanging around—like a fondness for soda or other sugary and/or caffeinated beverages—it will get rid of them, and far easier than if you tried to eliminate the habit through sheer will. If you have to hit 100 ounces of water, it will push off that midmorning latte or afternoon Diet Coke. (And honestly, the lack of energy you thought you needed caffeine to combat is likely due to dehydration, at least in part.) My only exceptions to the rule are plain sparkling water and green tea. Concentrate on getting your 100 ounces *first*, and once you get there, if you still want your diet soda, go for it.

Putting real water in the mix, every day, will make you feel like a different person. A few years ago, one of the women in a corporate weight-loss program I was running was doing everything right with her diet and exercise, but was drinking barely any water. She'd hit a plateau in her weight loss, and one week we made drinking more water her only goal. She aimed for the 100 ounces and came *skipping* into our meeting the following week. She said she felt like a completely new woman. She was glowing, her skin looked clearer, and her energy levels were through the roof. This one change, on top of her newly formed healthy food and exercise habits, made all the difference. She saw a weight loss that week after struggling for several without a drop on the scale.

THE HABIT OF HYDRATION

We have talked a lot (and will talk a lot more) about how our modern environment makes wellness more difficult. If 75 percent of the US population is walking around dehydrated, there is something seriously wrong. Unlike in many other parts of the world, clean water is freely available—if you are reading this book, I'll bet access to water is not your problem. So what is? Well, for one thing, we are so crazy busy in our overscheduled lives that we have become disconnected from what we are feeling in any given moment. We are focused on our to-do lists, not our bodies, and rarely take the time to pause and notice we are thirsty, much less stop, get up, and pour a glass of water. And, as a culture, we have created the habit of *not* drinking water. We drink caffeinated, sugary beverages once or twice a day, and often nothing else. Look, I won't begrudge you a caffeinated beverage if you drink your water. I love my coffee . . . but while the surge of caffeine in my veins gives a temporary burst of energy, it is also dehydrating,

THE GAME CHANGER FOR CHARLES BARKLEY

Every March, Charles Barkley heads into the toughest part of his year. As a March Madness commentator, his work gets incredibly intense as the basketball tournament heats up. Not only are there seemingly endless games to watch and dissect, there are seemingly endless new faces and up-and-coming talents for Charles to study and get to know. He is in the studio from midmorning until well past midnight every day—and when he's not in the studio, he's likely in a hotel room far from home watching and studying games and taking radio interviews over the phone. In our first year working together he knew that this period, with its long hours and the tempting food choices surrounding him, would be one of his biggest challenges. We wrote up a special March Madness game plan. It involved asking to have healthier meal options available in the studio and having a few meals delivered in. We focused on making sure he ate a solid breakfast in the hotel room, and had him bring single-serve snacks to the studio to serve as bridges between meals. Charles had a good first week but struggled during the second. We talked through his days again and discovered he was sometimes drinking up to *seven* diet sodas in the evening hours to keep himself alert and awake. He insisted he was so sluggish and tired that he needed them. Unfortunately, all that caffeine meant that by the time he got back to the hotel at night he was jittery and wired. Unable to fall asleep, he found himself indulging in late-night snacks from the minibar. The lack of sleep only made him more exhausted the next evening—and more likely to grab another soda for energy.

We promptly emptied out his minibar and filled it with yogurts and fresh fruit, and I went to work on his water consumption. He was not to drink a single soda until after he had a large bottle of water. Then he could have one diet soda, but before each additional one he had to drink another bottle of water. This reduced his diet soda consumption dramatically. The effect of this was so shockingly positive for him that he began replacing *all* of the soda with water— the water kept him more consistently energized than the caffeine did, and when he was done for the night he was able to fall right to sleep.

That year, for the first time in his career as a commentator, Charles lost weight rather than gaining it during the madness of March Madness.

---

and if you are having coffee in lieu of water, you'll actually have *less* energy over the course of the day, not more.

So, you've accepted that in order to make any real progress toward managing your weight, you must make hydration a priority. Unfortunately, as easy as this may sound, you will not "just remember to drink more water." It isn't your habit to do so. When I work with clients to create this habit, it turns out to be a surprisingly complex one. Most people don't "forget to eat" for more than a meal—you may forget to stop for lunch when work is hectic, but by late afternoon you don't need help to realize you are hungry. And yet plenty of people can get through a whole day never taking in more than a glass or two of liquid. How do you begin to cultivate the awareness of thirst, encourage trying water before you reach for food, and just generally get people to do something that often fails to enter their minds at all?

You rely on the habit loop of trigger▸routine▸reward. You get serious about *triggering* the intake of water at moments that are *consistent* and *stable*.

I worked hard on this with a corporate group in New York City. We created a culture of hydration. I gave each person a "gift" of a big, blue twenty-four-ounce tumbler, and then urged them to set alarms on their phones to remind them to refill those tumblers at intervals throughout the day. I gave the tumblers to every single employee, hoping that just seeing the giant tumbler on someone else's desk would "trigger" them to remember to refill their own. I encouraged everyone to bring their freshly filled tumbler to the meeting each week—and guzzle down the entire thing before leaving the forty-five-minute session. Every member set an individualized alarm on their phone that went off approximately as they entered the building, to trigger a new routine of filling their tumbler immediately upon getting into work. This was simple, but very effective, and it wasn't long before employees automatically headed to fill their tumblers as soon as they walked into the building. This is how you make change work: by systematically identifying potential triggers and creating new routines.

I love working on the habit of drinking more water. It provides a concrete opportunity to develop your habit formation skills without the emotions attached to food-related habits. It exposes the intricacies of a seemingly simple statement like, "I am going to drink more water," yet the possible triggers, new routines required, and rewards are all straightforward and easy to grasp. In my years at Weight Watchers, when someone was literally about to quit, I would often ask them if they could give me *one more week*, just one. In that week, their only job was to focus on drinking water. They invariably returned seven days later with an improved outlook, improved results, and renewed energy. Today, whenever a client gets discouraged, I take them back to "water only." Why? Because by narrowing your focus to being successful at just one thing—especially when that one thing doesn't require much in the way of overcoming temptation or inertia—you inevitably end up with a sense of accomplishment and ability.

If you are trying to lose weight and start to feel like you "just can't do it anymore," the reason is usually the same: it has become too complex, whether because your life has become suddenly more complicated, because you are trying to do too much at once, or because you are suffering from decision fatigue and simply need a break. Drop back to one essential pillar for a bit and you will be fine. "But Liz," I hear you say, "there is no way I will lose weight if I eat anything I want and just commit to drinking my water!" Try it. I have seen it work many times with people who insist they are ready to give up. Why? Because they really do *want* to lose weight. Even the small action of focusing on water intake *proves* that they want to lose

HYDRATION HELPERS

It's true: Water can get boring. That's why I recommend doing whatever you can to make it easy and fun. Get a bottle or tumbler that makes you happy to look at. Lots of people find it easier to drink water when it is really cold, so load up your tumbler with ice cubes. Keep sliced lemons or limes on hand (they store well in the freezer) to add some flavor, or try using an infuser to make flavored waters and keep them in your fridge! I include sparkling water in my guidelines specifically because it can go a long way in helping you break a soda habit and make it feel like you are having something a little more fun. I rely on seltzer with lime as my go-to first drink at parties and restaurants. It looks like I am having a drink so nobody bothers me about whether I am drinking or not, and it hydrates me prior to consuming any (dehydrating!) alcohol.

Seasonal changes can also be a challenge. In the colder months, you won't be as naturally attracted to drinking water. This is why I've included green tea. Hot water with lemon is better than it sounds, and while you'll have to count the carbs, steamed milk can help you stay hydrated in winter if you start really struggling to get your water in.

Obviously, I want you *drinking* water to get hydrated. But hydration is so important, there's no reason you shouldn't consider it when you're thinking about what to eat as well. The foods below all have high water content (and you'll notice they're mostly *very* low in carbs). If you're having a really hard time getting your 100 ounces in, adding these foods is a great "baby step" you can take toward your target:

1. Cucumber (96 percent water)
2. Iceberg lettuce (95 percent water)
3. Tomatoes (94 percent water)
4. Bell peppers (93 percent water)
5. Cauliflower (92 percent water)
6. Watermelon (91 percent water)
7. Spinach (91 percent water)
8. Baby carrots (90 percent water)
9. Broccoli (90 percent water)
10. Grapefruit (90 percent water)

weight. While they are making themselves proud via their success with water, they are also setting in motion a cycle of good choices that builds confidence and has its own momentum. They don't feel as hungry and their bodies are happier and those healthy choices begin to seem easier. Weight loss is full of intricate interconnections, but there are some simple things that simply work.

There is one stumbling block to developing this habit that isn't discussed much in diet or wellness books. Sometimes clients get really annoyed with me about it: "Liz, you didn't tell me I would become obsessed with locating bathrooms!" It will get better once your body adjusts, but yes, drinking more water does mean heading for the bathroom more than you're used to (especially if you've been chronically dehydrated!), and you will need to be aware of your consumption of water throughout the day in terms of your schedule— if you have back-to-back meetings every Tuesday, for instance, you might want to plan for a bathroom stop in between them. My client Sandy, who has a two-hour train commute to and from work, had to become strategic about when she drank her water in the morning . . . and when she stopped drinking it before jumping on the train home. She set a timer to remind her to fill her tumbler and begin drinking as soon as she walked into the office, and another to remind her to stop drinking around 3 PM. She also trained herself to hit the bathroom right as she left the building after work. Yes, building this habit will change your routine—on the plus side, getting up from your desk more often is good for you (we'll talk about this more in the chapter on movement)!

BOTTOMS UP!

The habit of hydration is simple, but not easy! This is where I see so many folks fail: they set the "goal" of drinking more water without any plan in place. Use the tools you have developed in previous targets to build this habit. Use the Habit Change Key, suggestions from the Habit Library at the end of this chapter, or whatever planning tools you have found work best for you. Identify the things that are likely to stand in your way, and think through your strategy before you begin. Then get ready to be shocked by how much better you feel!

HABIT LIBRARY

1. Place a glass of ice water next to your bed at night to drink upon waking in the morning.
2. Purchase reusable water bottles or tumblers for home and work.
3. Place a sticky note on the door to remind you to take your water bottle with you when leaving the house.
4. Drink one full glass of water before every meal.
5. Set up a trigger that reminds you to drink water throughout the day (alarm on phone, calendar notice, sticky note).
6. Make a batch of flavored ice cubes.
7. Set an alarm on your phone to remind you to stop drinking water two to three hours before bedtime so you can sleep through the night without needing the bathroom.
8. Drink one glass of water before drinking any alcohol.
9. Drink one glass of water in between every alcoholic beverage.
10. Try making a large batch of flavored water.
11. Slice lemons and limes to keep on hand to put in water and seltzer.
12. Make a seasonal shift to warm beverages in colder months.
13. Drop one caffeinated beverage per day and replace with water.
14. Remove soda from your diet.
15. Add hydrating foods to every meal (see list above).
16. Map out the best bathrooms throughout your day.
17. Set a case of water by the door. Leave a sticky note at eye level to remind you to grab one as you leave.
18. Drink a full glass of water first thing when sitting down to a restaurant meal.
19. Ask a friend to be your "water buddy," reminding you and working with you to remember to drink water.
20. Start a water challenge at work or at home. Challenge coworkers or your family to drink 100 ounces every day.
21. When hunger or a craving strikes, try drinking water first, then reevaluate.
22. Start taking water with you when you are out shopping or running errands—the air in stores is often dry, and it will help you avoid impulse-buying a beverage.
23. Experiment with green teas.
24. Try out an infuser bottle.
25. If this target is just not happening for you, try adding just ten extra ounces—and then another ten extra next week.

TARGETS
3 AND 4

EXERCISE

AND MOVEMENT

Chapter 6

EXERCISE THERAPY

E veryone is always telling me how "nice" I am. I guess I have one of those faces—I look like the (nice) mom in a juice commercial. And you know what? It's true; I *am* nice! But in this chapter I am serving up some tough love.

Can you lose weight without exercising? Absolutely. Will it be the lasting weight loss I want for you and know you want for yourself? Not a chance. And guess what? The reason I want you to exercise has nothing to do with burning calories. Nope, from my perspective, exercise is the magical secret sauce that teaches you what you are made of. It shows you that you are stronger than you know. It opens your eyes to the fact that anything you want to achieve is absolutely yours. It erodes self-doubt and builds the confidence you will need to take this program forward long term. It is a nonnegotiable part of this formula. Period. Weight loss is a mind game more than anything else, and exercise is the tool that will get your mind in the right place. You can roll your eyes at this, or panic and say, "But I *can't*!" But the truth is, I'm right, and you *can*! It's simply a matter of looking at exercise from a new perspective and coming up with a unique workout strategy that fits you and your life. In this chapter, I'll help you figure out what activities you enjoy, and show you how to begin a workout program by starting where you are.

EXERCISE IS ABOUT CHANGING YOUR BRAIN, NOT YOUR BODY

There's no doubt about it: To be healthy, we should all be working out several times a week, to build muscle mass and strengthen the cardiovascular system. It is also true that exercise burns calories and can reshape the body. However, I have always had a very different take on why exercise is an essential piece of the weight-loss puzzle. Exercise is difficult. It challenges us to schedule and think ahead. It forces us to put ourselves first. Most importantly of all, it makes us *uncomfortable.* The physical, mental, and emotional discomfort that you experience during exercise is the key training you will need to be able to make difficult food choices, to manage the emotions that send you running to the fridge, to face all the other discomforts and frustrations that will undoubtedly occur over the course of the weight-loss process. It will be your training ground. Changing your life requires understanding how to push through difficult times, and for most of us, there is no other place to flex those muscles regularly than during exercise. The world we live in offers us endless ways to avoid discomfort. We have a never-ending stream of distractions and lifestyles that ensure most of us do little to no physical labor. Getting our heart rate up feels strange or even scary; sweating is something to be avoided at all costs. And avoiding things we do not like is easy: We have an array of conveniences that allow us to avoid saying "no" to ourselves, or learning to manage our feelings of anxiety, fear, and frustration. Exercise will force you to deal with these feelings. Get to know them intimately. Understand that they do not last forever, and you have the strength to handle them in a healthy way.

To this day, I have at least one moment in every exercise session when I think to myself: *I want to quit.* Sometimes it comes halfway through, sometimes before I am even out the door or have the DVD playing. I am guessing this is familiar to all of us. It's a little voice whispering in my ear, trying to convince me that I don't have time or I'm too tired or I should be doing something else instead. As I gained more and more experience with exercise, I began to recognize that I could count on this voice showing up every time, and realized that this was exactly why exercise was so important: I began to see exercise as an opportunity to train my brain against those negative thoughts and feelings. I also began to notice that these were the same types of thoughts that popped up throughout the day in other

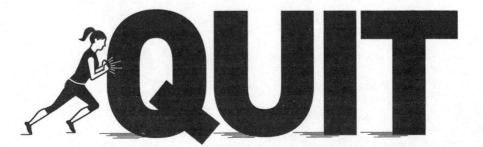

situations, and that practicing pushing through these thoughts in the exercise arena was paying off. Suddenly I was beginning to be able to handle difficult food choices more easily, and found I could face stressful moments in general with less anxiety. I'd often fought the urge to "quit" my food plan, but with the added practice of pushing those "quitting thoughts" away in exercise, they became easier to push away everywhere.

I was, simply, getting stronger. Negative thoughts and feelings bubble up all day long in our minds, like a radio playing in the background. Before I became consistent with exercise, it seemed like the radio's messages were controlling me—my moods, my willpower, my decisions. With exercise, I found I could turn the radio's volume down and focus on what was important to me.

YOU DON'T GET A COOKIE

I just said exercise is a vital part of the weight-loss equation, but at the same time, I want you to divorce your exercise practice from your weight. Exercise is in your program as a training ground, an expansion tool. It is there for increased energy and greater strength both physically and emotionally. It is *not* there to "burn off" what you eat. You can't outrun your fork.

In a thirty- to forty-five-minute exercise session you might—*might*—burn 350 to 500 calories. In food, that is the equivalent of a cupcake, or maybe a handful of Oreos. I don't know about you, but I can scarf either one of those down in about two minutes. Faster if I'm really hungry (like

I might be after, say, exercising). Those just are not numbers that work in your favor. Two minutes of reward for forty-five minutes of work? It makes no sense to think of it that way—you will end up frustrated and resentful. What's more, most people consistently *over*estimate how much they've exercised while *under*estimating the amount of food they consume. So my rule is that exercise simply isn't currency: it doesn't "buy" you anything. Stop giving yourself permission to eat more because you exercised that day (unless you are well beyond the target of 100 minutes). And let's all be honest: when we use exercise to buy ourselves extra food, it is rarely baby carrots and apple slices. We use it to get another glass of wine or a slice of cake. You can't kid a kidder. This is how I trained for and ran a marathon and gained weight in the process . . . it was not muscle weight, friends! Eat the cake or have that drink, but do not "excuse"

WORDS OF LIZDOM

Doing things that make you feel virtuous, like getting your exercise in, can set the tone for your entire day. Once you feel that sense of pride (let's be real, almost *smugness*) you will want to protect it, and the decisions that follow are more likely to be in line with your goals.

it away with exercise, because there is no need to. The cake or wine didn't make you a bad person. It isn't shameful. It just is. I can't tell you how many times I have said to clients, "It's only food, you didn't kill anybody!" Remember, guilt and shame actually drive the reward center, creating a toxic feedback loop. Stay aware of all the ways in which the mind tells us we can "erase" our choices, opting instead for looking them straight in the eye without judgment.

So, step back from your old ways of thinking about exercise. Give yourself, and exercise, a clean slate. This is not going to feel the same at all, believe me. I spent years overexercising, trying endlessly to outrun my fork. I was resentful and felt like a failure. When I stopped looking at exercise as a way to burn calories or erase some "shameful" or "guilty" decision I'd made the day before, my attitude about it transformed. I began to relish rewards that had nothing to do with a weight-loss goal I was hoping to reach weeks or months in the future, but instead were immediate, in-the-moment successes: my abilities growing and the pride I felt as a result; the increased energy that day and better sleep that night; my more relaxed response to stressful situations.

Make exercise about achieving physical goals, about running farther or faster, about learning to dance or lifting heavier weights. See these accomplishments for what they are rather than burying them under food choices. This will change your life. Exercise is a measurable and easy way to build confidence in yourself—and I absolutely guarantee, from years of experience with clients, you are stronger and more capable than you know. Seeing clients surprise themselves in this way is probably the most rewarding part of my job. Use exercise to show yourself that by consistently taking small steps forward, you can do what seems impossible.

DEFINING THE TARGET

I am asking you to build to at least 100 minutes each week of moderate to high-intensity exercise. Your exercise minutes should include some muscle strengthening. Many people, especially women, are surprised to discover that they find weight lifting extremely rewarding, and for those of us with frantic schedules, it is a great way to get a high-intensity workout in a short period of time. Exercise, as we are defining it here, is something that actually gets your heart rate up and stresses the muscles. Exercise is a specific, planned, purposeful physical activity that you do with the intention of acquiring greater fitness or other health benefits. It is not the same thing as "movement," which is why I have separated these concepts into two targets. "Movement" may include planned walks you take specifically in order to reach your movement target, but it also includes the activities we do throughout the day that just happen to require us to move, like housework, gardening, and climbing stairs. Examples of exercise include running, weight lifting, biking . . . and yes, yoga and even walking.

Each of us will take aim at this target from our own unique starting point, depending upon our fitness level. Some of you may already be devoted runners or gym goers; others may not be exercising at all. I love walking as a "gateway drug" for those who are just starting out, and it is a great way to stay active while recovering from injury. I have seen people lose hundreds of pounds with walking as their only form of exercise. The key to this target— and every target—is giving yourself permission to start from wherever you are now.

When I coach someone in beginning a walking program for their form of exercise, I encourage them to adopt a few requirements, and I'd suggest you adopt these as well. First, I want you to schedule a specific time for your walking. This should be different than your walk to the train or bus or car. This is time set aside for you to really focus on challenging yourself. Secondly, *do* challenge yourself: Try hills when a flat terrain becomes easy, or time yourself and work on increasing distance or speed. Get your arms pumping and heart rate up. Feel a little burn in your legs and flush in your cheeks!

Now let me be transparent. The Center for Disease Control (CDC) recommends 150 minutes of exercise a week. I definitely agree with those numbers, and I'd love to get you there and higher—pretty much everyone I have ever worked with needed to "up" the amount of exercise they were doing. But what isn't realistic isn't sustainable, and what isn't sustainable is pretty much pointless. The first step is building the habit, and the truth is that for most people, "exercise" is a dirty word. In focus groups at Weight Watchers, we found that the word "exercise" had such negative connotations for people that the program ultimately banished the word from the curriculum completely, training leaders to always say "activity" instead. I am not going to do that here. You're a grown-up, and I'm pretty sure that you know when you're exercising. But this chapter, and the book as a whole, is trying to teach you that starting small *works*. Small, manageable goals are what we are wired for. One hundred minutes works out to twenty minutes five times a week. It is doable, easy to remember, and enough exercise to see significant results and benefits.

To get started, you need to look honestly at where you are now—how much exercise are you *really* getting, every week? Some of you may already be hitting the 100-minute target. If so, use the strategies outlined in this chapter to add minutes. If you are at zero, don't feel overwhelmed—start with twenty minutes for the week, or ten minutes a day, or whatever feels doable to you. Pick a number you *know* you can hit consistently, and build the behavior, then build it up. By adding even one minute each week, you can end up running marathons—I have a client who did just that! More importantly, before you know it you'll have formed a nonnegotiable exercise habit. Working toward more exercise slowly, in achievable, measured steps, will ensure that you don't get injured, that you banish any negative feelings about exercise, and that you continue to grow and get stronger at a steady and sustainable pace.

UNPACK YOUR FEELINGS ABOUT EXERCISE

Take some time to briefly jot down your earliest memories and experiences with exercise. Uncover where and when you made decisions about what you were capable of and what exercise was like for you.

Then, write out how you will change your perceptions and assumptions about exercise as you move forward.

_____

_____

_____

_____

_____

_____

_____

_____

_____

_____

_____

Now that you've thought about your past experiences with exercise and what you can learn from them, open your mind a bit on the subject. Maybe you hate gyms but have always wanted to learn to salsa dance. Maybe you know a gym with free childcare and would try anything for a toddler-free hour. Maybe you loved playing soccer when you were in college, or remember an amazing afternoon hike from your honeymoon. Could you find a way to make exercise something fun? Take a minute to assess your current relationship with exercise, using the questions below:

THE EXERCISE EXERCISE

I *consistently* exercise _____ times a week.

My favorite type of exercise is _____.

If I were to explore a new type of exercise, it would likely be

_____.

To begin exploring that new exercise, three small steps I could take would be:

1. _____

2. _____

3. _____

The thing I find most challenging about exercise is

_____.

The thing I like most about exercise is _____

_____

_____.

WHERE THERE'S A *WILL*: MAKING IT WORK, STEP BY STEP

Informational learning is gaining knowledge about a topic by gathering information about it—for instance, reading an article on all the health benefits of regular exercise. *Transformational learning* is taking action and doing, discovering along the way what you don't know and problem solving as you go. Guess which one is more effective? Yes, exercise will absolutely make you happier and healthier in a million ways you have probably already heard about a million times, but I'm not going to bore you further with all the reasons you *should* exercise. In fact, let's remove the word "should" from our vocabulary. Let's replace it with "will." And when you say that you "will" do something, make sure that you *actually do it*. One of the most important benefits of learning to set achievable, personalized goals, goals that make sense for our lives, is that it allows us to neutralize whatever feelings of shame or failure we might be carrying from previous attempts at weight loss by rebuilding our sense of integrity. As we begin to follow through on the things we promise ourselves, we regain some of the trust and confidence we lost by not honoring our promises to ourselves in the past. It's time to get out of your own way, stop telling yourself how you feel about exercise, and allow transformation to happen.

Today, you have an advantage you didn't have before! You can set yourself up for success by applying all of your new habit-formation strategies. You understand that this one habit involves many smaller habit changes and life tasks, all rolled up in the deceptively simple statement "I'm going to start exercising." Planning to start tomorrow? Great! Here are a few questions:

- Will you exercise in the morning, or wait until after work?
- If you are exercising in the morning, what time will you need to get up?
- Will you eat breakfast first?
- If you are exercising after work, how will this affect dinner?
- What will you wear to exercise?
- Will you shower after?
- Do you need any special gear, like different shoes, a sports bra, weights, or a yoga mat?

Let's take my client Kelly as an example. Kelly knew she "should" exercise. She also knew that, due to an injury, she couldn't do anything high impact, so she decided that she would join a local gym and start aerobic swimming classes. Weeks went by and she simply couldn't get it done. When she met with me, she expressed her frustration. "Why do I continually avoid this?" she moaned. "Something is wrong with me!" She was angry at herself for not "taking action."

I told her she may as well have decided to climb Mount Everest. If we look at what Kelly had decided to do—join a local gym and start aerobic swimming classes—we can see it had several actions and steps involved. Just joining a gym is intimidating enough! To do even that, she needed to research gyms to see which had swimming pools and classes, visit the gym she chose, and do all the paperwork involved with signing up for a membership. We needed to separate out the various parts of Kelly's goal and divide them into actionable tasks she could easily accomplish, one by one. So, in our first week of focusing on exercise, we actually did no exercise at all. Instead, we focused on and set goals around the "prep steps" that would make exercise possible in her life. This is something that most people miss. For any big behavior modification

Lower the bar of success until you can step over it. This will create the momentum you need to roll forward with your new habit.

like exercise, there is likely an entire universe of decisions and tasks that need to happen first. Those "prep" tasks were just as important for Kelly as the exercise itself—they were teaching her how to properly manage any new behavior change so that it is more likely to become a lasting one. In Kelly's first week, her tasks included research on local gyms, gym visits, and joining a gym. That was more than enough with a full-time job and three kids! She handily accomplished those tasks, and guess what? *Because* she accomplished them and did what she said she would do, she felt great. That happiness and pride got her excited for the following week's tasks and even inspired her to make better food choices. In short, it gave her confidence and momentum, and *that* is transformational.

Kelly assigned herself three tasks in the first week. Like most of us, she has a busy life, and so in order to make these tasks happen, we had to make sure they had a space in her schedule and were triggered—otherwise they would be forgotten or pushed out by other demands on her time. We pulled out her calendar and set aside blocks in her day throughout the week to work on her tasks—to research gyms, call friends who worked out there, visit the facilities herself—and set reminders on her phone as triggers. We leveraged the familiar habit loop of trigger, routine, reward. By backing up and examining the tasks associated with a complicated behavior change, Kelly could trigger those tasks and then reap the rewards of moving her goal forward and feeling good about herself. Could she have pushed it and done more that first week? Sure! But isn't there a saying that goes "do what you always did and get what you always got"? In the past, Kelly would have pushed (and likely failed) by putting too much on her plate. That is likely your old habit, too, your old routine. I know it was mine. And though I wasn't really aware of it, that old routine was powerful because it was *also* getting me something I wanted, which was to

GETTING OLDER, GETTING STRONGER

We should actually be exercising *more* as we age—not less. The problem is that as we get older, we accumulate more and more responsibilities that compete for our time. In my twenties I had no kids and worked at a pizza parlor. I had loads of time to do the step aerobics classes I loved so much in the early nineties! Now I have a career I'm passionate about, two kids, a husband, and a house to tend to. The majority of my clients have similar stories: Exercise has fallen by the wayside, and they can't figure out how to fit it back in. To find the hidden opportunities in their hectic days, they need to take the time to examine them and plan accordingly. Their lives have changed, and they need to adjust.

The other thing that changes is our bodies themselves. One of my first high-profile clients at Weight Watchers was Katie Couric. Katie had a history as a gymnast, so she didn't mind exercise, and she was already eating pretty well. She was perplexed by why she was beginning to gain weight when her routine hadn't changed. Of course, this was the problem—the Pilates and yoga she'd been doing three to four times a week for years was no match for a slowing metabolism. We spent an entire summer attending every kind of exercise class you can find in NYC—even Zumba, laughing at ourselves in the mirror as we tried to keep up—but it was when she tried cycling that Katie was hooked. With this more vigorous exercise, she soon started to see results.

Another issue I see is that, sometimes, we stubbornly hold on to a type of exercise that no longer works for us because we have new physical limitations or injuries. Maybe 20-year-old you loved running, but 40-year-old you has a bad knee. Yes, you should be getting more exercise as you age, but you may have to modify your workouts before they can increase. The good news is that research proves we can be just as strong well into our seventies as we were in our forties—*if* we keep ourselves fit.

avoid establishing an exercise habit at all—because it was too hard. This way, I could be the victim: I tried and failed, and I could throw up my hands and stay put, continuing my comfortably familiar life unchanged. The next week, Kelly's tasks included checking the schedule of classes and timing the walk to her workplace from the gym. She also needed to get herself a swimsuit, goggles, and flip-flops. Finally, in the third week, she scheduled her first session, packed her gym bag to leave by the door, and made it to class. Her only goal was to stay in the pool for the entire time—if she needed to sit out an exercise or two that was fine, as long as she stayed until the end of class. Kelly knew she was out of shape at this point, and it was important that she avoid getting so sore or overtired that the experience became one she dreaded repeating. Kelly's goal then became to get to just that one class for each of the next three weeks. When she was feeling stronger, we layered on a second class. By then, exercise was beginning to feel familiar—the habit was taking root.

EXERCISE ENEMIES

Everyone has had the experience of starting an exercise program with the best of intentions, only to find themselves derailed and discouraged. Let's talk about some of the problems you might run into, and what to do about them.

Boredom

It's easy to get stuck in a rut. I watch as clients start out loving a particular exercise—like kickboxing—so much that they decide to do it every single time they work out, only to get bored and ruin it for themselves! Understand that you may need a "repertoire" of workout choices to pull from. I have an array of exercise options that I vary based on factors like mood, weather, and time. Below you'll find my repertoire, and a chance for you to think about your own.

LIZ'S EXERCISE REPERTOIRE

RAINY OR SNOWY DAY: Work out in my basement with exercise DVD or program via streaming services or YouTube.

TOTALLY UNMOTIVATED DAY: Get myself to a class to be surrounded by energy and people. (This pushes and inspires me to see it through!)

GORGEOUS WEATHER DAY: Take a run outside or do an outdoor activity—like swimming—that I love.

GOOD WEATHER ON A WEEKEND WHEN MY HUSBAND IS AVAILABLE: Work out together or play a game of tennis.

TRAVELING: Get on the treadmill in the hotel gym, even if it's just for thirty minutes.

TRAVELING WITH EXTRA TIME: Try a local exercise class or outdoor running route.

YOUR EXERCISE REPERTOIRE

Rainy or snowy day: _____

Totally unmotivated day: _____

Gorgeous weather day: _____

Traveling: _____

Traveling with extra time: _____

Others, specific to your life:

_____ : _____

_____ : _____

Setting Overly Aggressive Goals
(To Perform Activities You Don't Even Like)

I had a friend who hated getting wet, but decided that since swimming is so good for you, she'd start exercising by swimming laps for half an hour five mornings a week. This plan failed miserably (of course) on the first morning, when my out-of-shape friend, exhausted and discouraged, pulled herself out of the pool after six laps and headed to a donut shop to smother her sorrows in pastry. You wouldn't think I'd have to say this, but here I go: Choose an activity you *enjoy*! Jennifer Hudson is not a fan of working out, but she loves basketball. She uses playing basketball with her husband and kids as a way to fit exercise in—while having fun. And just because you like something doesn't mean starting small goes out the window! Liking hockey or biking doesn't mean it's realistic to strap on your skates or helmet seven days a week.

Lack of Support

The same things that make exercise so important—the discomfort and growth it inspires—make it one of the harder targets for many. Find people in your life (or put some there!) who support your efforts in a way that is effective and meaningful to *you*. Be clear about the balance of encouragement and tough love you need, and identify someone—a friend, an online buddy, your spouse—who will push you, but not too far too fast; someone who will cheer you on, but not give you an easy out. Sustaining an exercise habit is easier with friends who will meet in the park at 6 AM for a hike or brave a local boot camp with you. If you're on your own right now, look for classes or groups or running clubs that give you an opportunity to connect with others, whether in person or online. Surround yourself with people who will support the lifestyle you're building.

The Scale

Yet another reason to divorce exercise from weight loss is that as you begin to be more active, you may notice some funky things happening on the scale. When clients begin an exercise regimen, I often challenge them to weigh themselves every day for thirty days. (I've included a chart at the end of the chapter if you'd like to try this yourself.) I do this to show them that exercise can really mess with the numbers. I urge clients not to put too much stock in what effect exercise has on their weight, and find other ways to measure progress, for instance by taking measurements with a tape measure or using a body composition scale that measures changes in body-fat percentage. Physiologically, when you begin any new exercise routine (especially if that routine makes you sore!) your body will hold on to water around the muscles to soothe and help heal them. Working a muscle creates microscopic tears in its fibers, and just as when you burn your hand on the stove and it puffs up and gets red, when you tear down muscle to build it up, the body reacts as it would to any other injury—with inflammation and a rush of fluid to the area. I've seen this fact send so many people off the deep end over the course of my career—they finally get themselves to the gym, and then their weekly weigh-in rolls around and they've "gained!" Their weight loss hadn't actually stalled or reversed, they were just bloated and inflamed. Some would give up before they had the chance to see that weight slide right off again.

Another issue is that somewhat misleading saying you've probably heard your whole life: "Muscle weighs more than fat." Of course, one pound of muscle is exactly equal to one pound of fat, but if you have two cardboard boxes of the same size, one filled with muscle and one filled with fat, the one with muscle will indeed weigh more because a pound of muscle fills up less space than a pound of fat. A (less gruesome) visual that works well is to envision one pound of popcorn kernels (muscle) vs. one pound of popped popcorn (fat). Muscle is smooth and packed tightly, whereas fat is fluffy and takes up much more room. Our goal is to replace popped popcorn with popcorn kernels. Now you can understand why you might see a dramatic shift in someone's appearance when they begin working out, yet they may not lose any weight or may even gain some. Just recently I upped my exercise in time and intensity. I was so glad I had a body composition scale! I started out with a body-fat percentage in the 35 percent range. Over the past six months I've taken that down to 28 percent. My clothes are fitting better, they're even

Another Benefit of Building Muscle. Muscle burns more calories than fat, just by existing—by gaining muscle you actually raise your metabolic rate. But in order to build that lean muscle, we need extra protein. The recommended daily intake of protein for adults is about 25 to 30 grams at each meal. Most Americans are not hitting those numbers. Luckily, reducing your carb intake forces you to choose more foods rich in protein and healthy fats. Include protein at every meal, and know that protein sources rich in the amino acid leucine seem to stimulate muscle synthesis more than others. Leucine-rich proteins include milk, whey, tuna, beef, chicken, soy, peanuts, and eggs.

a little loose, yet I weigh *more* than I did six months ago! The point is, the scale is just one measurement tool. You can also use compliments, clothing, measurements, and body composition to gauge progress.

Lack of Planning

This is the biggie, which is why we've spent most of this chapter discussing it already! Take time to think through your week and where you might fit 100 minutes of exercise into your life. When we actually look at what we are doing each hour of the day—which we'll do more formally in the next chapter—we can usually find slots of time where it's possible to squeeze in exercise, even fifteen minutes at a time. Perhaps mindless Facebook scrolling is sucking out thirty minutes after work you could use to take a walk, or there's an hour of TV at night you could lift weights while watching. Figure out what you need to do before you begin and create a specific, concrete goal. Remember Kelly. Use her example, and all the habit-formation tools you've developed so far, to break your goal into steps and make a plan that will ensure success.

BABY STEPS

Speaking of Kelly, funnily enough, over the weeks we worked together, she often complained about how easy it all was. She felt impatient and worried it "wouldn't work" my way. She wanted to feel the familiar pain and frustration she had so many times before when attempting to begin an exercise routine. She wanted it to hurt! "How well did *that* work?" I asked her. Not so great, she had to admit. She also admitted that it was awfully nice to be keeping promises to herself and moving steadily toward her goal *every single week*. It doesn't matter if you get to the gym that first week if by week four you have no intention of going back. As we've discussed throughout this book, it is more important to build something lasting than to get off to a running start. We understand this in so many other areas of our lives, but when it comes to weight loss and fitness, we abandon our common sense. You likely didn't get to where you are in your career without many incremental, carefully thought-out steps. You allowed yourself to grow and learn and change. I like to think of myself as the baby I once was. As I was learning to walk, no one ridiculed me for taking only one wobbly step, shoving me over because I wasn't learning fast enough! We are patient as we watch our plants grow from seedlings to tomatoes over the summer months, but we aren't patient with ourselves. You should never feel demoralized and defeated by exercise. Be patient, and let yourself grow.

HABIT LIBRARY

1. Go to the gym (no workout required!) just to create the habit of getting there.
2. Set out your workout clothes at night to trigger you to exercise in the morning.
3. Ask a friend to join you for a run or an exercise class.
4. Sign up for a Fun Run or 3K. (This is a great thing to do with your kids!)
5. Buy a new pair of shoes.
6. Research exercise classes in your neighborhood.
7. Prepare a post-exercise snack to have on hand.
8. Try a new exercise DVD.
9. Try a streaming exercise service.
10. Buy new workout clothing.
11. Schedule your exercise a week ahead.
12. Pack a gym bag to leave at work with a full set of necessary gear.
13. If you usually exercise at night, try exercising first thing in the morning.
14. If you usually exercise in the morning, try exercising at night.
15. Join an online exercise community.
16. Add one-minute high-intensity cardio surges to your strength-training routine.
17. Exercise as a family.
18. Try a new sport.
19. Try a session with a personal trainer.
20. Add one minute to each workout in your week.
21. Add incline to your walk or run, whether on a machine or by choosing a hilly route.
22. Reduce rest time between sets.
23. Keep an exercise journal.
24. Share your workout on social media ("Today I . . .").
25. Increase your reps by five, or your weights by two pounds.

EXERCISE AND WEIGHT WORKSHEET

Once you have begun your new exercise routine, weigh in for thirty days straight to see how working out can affect the scale. Look at this as a science project, and regard your data without emotion.

DAY	DATE	WEIGHT	NOTES
1			
2			
3			
4			
5			
6			
7			
8			
9			
10			
11			
12			
13			
14			
15			
16			
17			
18			
19			
20			
21			
22			
23			
24			
25			
26			
27			
28			
29			
30			

Chapter 7

MOVE MORE

ey, Liz, didn't we cover this already? You just did an entire chapter on exercise, remember? Yup, I remember, but this chapter isn't about exercise, it's about *movement*. People tend to lump them together, but I have always viewed them separately—after all, they serve very different purposes. Exercise, remember, is a specific, planned, purposeful physical activity that gets your heart rate up and stresses the muscles. Movement, on the other hand, refers to our ordinary functional activity throughout the day—things like walking, doing housework, gardening, and climbing stairs. These essential movements have, little by little, been sucked out of our daily lives. Exercise is crucial for all the reasons we discussed in the last chapter, particularly as a mental training ground that builds your confidence and emotional stamina. However, to achieve sustainable, long-term weight loss (not to mention wellness), it is simply not enough to get to the gym for thirty to sixty minutes in the morning if we then spend the rest of the day mostly sitting down. It stunts metabolism, torpedoes bone density, and actually shortens our life span. Target 100 asks you to focus on exercise and movement as two distinct and equally important aspects of your program.

BUSY IS NOT THE SAME AS ACTIVE

You may have heard the saying "sitting is the new smoking." We'll talk about how they're alike later, but right now I want to focus on what makes them different. Smoking is a pretty obvious habit, one that's easy to recognize in ourselves. It is hard to miss the fact that you took out a cigarette and lit it. But what I can tell you from working with people from all walks of life is that no one is actually doing much walking: we simply don't realize how sedentary we've become. In fact, in surveys, 65 percent of American adults consider themselves "active," while actually, when observed, only about 5 percent would be classified this way.

We don't have a lot of ways to quantify how active we are in a day—the following chart uses steps as a measure of what "active" looks like.

👣 MY STEPS	HOW ACTIVE AM I?
< 5,000 STEPS	SEDENTARY
5,000 – 7,499 STEPS	UNDER ACTIVE
7,500 – 9,999 STEPS	SOMEWHAT ACTIVE
10,000 – 12,499	ACTIVE
> 12,500	HIGHLY ACTIVE

Take a minute, right now, to estimate your own activity level:

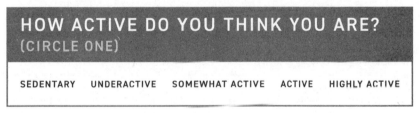

HOW ACTIVE DO YOU THINK YOU ARE?
(CIRCLE ONE)

SEDENTARY   UNDERACTIVE   SOMEWHAT ACTIVE   ACTIVE   HIGHLY ACTIVE

When I start working with a new client, I ask them to track their steps for a few days—either using their phone's step counter, a pedometer, or a wearable fitness tracker—*without* changing any of their routines. But before they start, I ask them to guess, approximately, how many steps they are getting in an average day. We write that number down and then I sit back and wait. It never fails: they come back *shocked*. The number they guessed is way off; they were sure they were so much more active than they actually are. It blows their minds to realize how out of touch they are with their own reality—they've heard the talk about sedentary lifestyles but didn't think it applied to them.

I have a personal, nonscience-based hypothesis about why this is. I think people feel—and are!—so "busy" that they actually believe they are on the move all the time. Unfortunately, studies paint a very different picture, showing that more than 60 percent of our waking hours are sedentary. Let's use my client Mary as an example: Mary has kids and a full-time job. She is *hectic* busy. She was certain she was getting at least 10,000 steps a day, but when she started tracking found that the number was closer to 5,000. Mary simply didn't realize that as busy as she was, our lifestyles have us sitting all day long: in trains, cars, and buses, at desks in front of computers, and on couches in front of TV screens. Below is Mary's day before we started adding activity. (Warning: May sound familiar.)

Wake up and get ready for work; drive to train station	500 steps
Train ride into the city, seated	0 steps
Walk to subway from train	750 steps
Walk from subway to work	750 steps
Work all day, in front of a computer, except when back and forth to meetings; lunch ordered in by assistant	500 steps
Return commute home—walk from work to subway, from subway to train, then sit on train	1,500 steps
Jump in car—spend the next two hours running kids to practices and picking up dinner at the local pizza place	500 steps
At home, wind down for the night; get kids to bed; clean up; then sit and watch TV until bedtime	1,000 steps
TOTAL FOR THE DAY:	**5,500 STEPS**

As you can see, Mary was excruciatingly busy. But not so active. She was dumbfounded to discover how little movement her day held, and despairing about where in her crazy schedule she would fit more in. To be as active as she'd thought she was, Mary would have to basically double her steps, and it's not like she had a bunch of free time to go and take long, leisurely walks.

Lack of movement has snuck up on us as a society pretty quickly. Even fifty years ago, the daily lives of most Americans were filled with small motions that have now been eliminated by "helpful" technologies. We have cell phones and computers, dishwashers and delivery. My husband calls it the "Blockbuster Effect." Back in the day, if you wanted to watch a movie from the comfort of your living room, you had to go to the video store, wander the aisles to browse the selection, and then make the return trip home. Today, not only is there no need to venture outside, you never have to leave the couch—just scroll through the streaming options with a remote or your ever-present smartphone. And this is just one example. Remember when we actually had to get up from our desks to talk to a colleague? To print something? Now we have email and chat applications, PDFs and e-signatures. Remember when we had to push carts through grocery stores, carry bags to the car, stand in the kitchen cooking dinner? Now we have grocery delivery and convenience foods. We have even begun eliminating the tiny amount of movement involved in typing—you can compose an email, send a text message, or perform an internet search using nothing but your voice! Unfortunately, Newton was on to something with his first law of motion: A body at rest tends to stay at rest. The more we sit, the harder it is to get up and move.

Another problem, one I've not only observed with clients but have seen from getting older myself, is that we naturally tend to slow down as we age. Year after year, we move less and less. I have even noticed that, now that my kids are old enough, I've started asking them to "go upstairs and get something for me" to avoid that climb to the second floor. Unfortunately, as I mentioned earlier, we should be moving more as we age, not less! The symptoms we think of as reasons for moving less with age—aches and pains, brittle bones—are all improved with movement and exercise! It is difficult to fight the natural tendencies and cultural ideas that plague us, but we need more movement each year.

SITTING SICKNESS

Why am I so concerned about this? For one thing, there are endless negative health effects from sitting too much. Over 10,000 studies conclude that prolonged sitting will reduce your life span and promote disease, *even if you exercise regularly*. (This is reason enough to separate exercise and movement, in my opinion!) What's more, many of

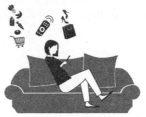

Technology has made our lives easier . . . and much less active. New apps and gadgets appear at an astounding rate; thanks to Amazon Echo and Google Home, even crossing the room to flip a light switch may soon be a thing of the past. Here are just a few examples of everyday opportunities for movement we've begun to opt out of in recent decades:

- Grocery shopping and food prep
- Shopping for clothing, shoes, furniture (and just about everything else)
- Getting up to change the channel on the TV, answer the phone, change a CD, or (remember this?) turn over a record
- Doctor visits for minor ailments (hello, eVisits!)
- Visiting libraries or browsing bookstores (hello, e-books!)
- Movies in theaters (my children are horrified to hear that long ago, it was the *only way to see them*) and, later, video rental
- Washing dishes by hand
- Walking because you don't have the car (multicar families are a fairly new development, after all)
- Mailing bills and letters, buying stamps, sending packages
- Banking

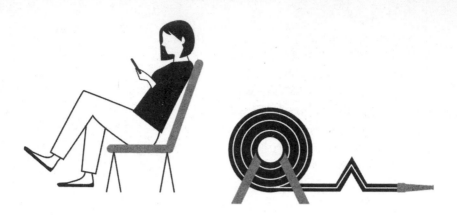

those effects directly impact weight loss. I explain the global effects of sitting to clients this way: when you are seated, your body is like a giant, bent garden hose.

Try running water through a bent hose—it flows half as fast. When you sit, your blood actually flows more slowly through your system. When blood flow is constricted, metabolism grinds to a screeching halt. Our bodies were literally designed for movement. When we sit for prolonged periods, we slow vital processes throughout the body, and what is scariest is that this can change the way our bodies function at a molecular and hormonal level. Here are just a few of the health problems linked to lack of consistent movement:

- **Diabetes.** Studies show that even one day of sitting can cause the pancreas to overproduce insulin, which, over time, may lead to the development of diabetes. In fact, those who sit for more than eight hours a day have a 90 percent increased risk of type 2 diabetes. In other words, their risk is doubled. Once I heard that statistic, I got very serious with my family about movement. I make my kids walk to and from school every day. It is just over a half mile each way, and we do it rain, shine, snow, or sleet. I am determined that they get some movement in before they start another day at their desks. Every other family is loading kids into a van or car as we walk past—I think the people in my neighborhood think I am a Mean Mom. I can live with that.
- **Cancer.** Cancers *love* a sedentary body. Prolonged sitting increases the risks of colon, breast, and endometrial cancers. The theory is that slowing blood flow also slows the production and circulation of the antioxidants that would otherwise fight these cancers off.
- **Heart disease.** When you're sitting, you burn less fat. Those extra fatty acids floating around in your bloodstream can clog your arteries, leading

to a greater risk of heart disease. Prolonged sitting also ups your risk for blood clots and circulatory problems.

- **Heartburn, acid reflux, and other digestive issues.** Remember the bent garden hose image? Just imagine what sitting does to the digestive tract and stomach. When we sit after meals, we compress the food in our abdomen, which slows digestion and can lead to heartburn, acid reflux, bloating, and constipation. There is a reason these ailments are on the rise. This is more than just a matter of discomfort—over the long term, heartburn and acid reflux can lead to bleeding ulcers and cancers of the esophagus and stomach. Amazingly, we've chosen to treat these symptoms with widespread use of medications like Prilosec, when the solution may be as simple as taking a fifteen-minute walk after each meal.
- **Musculoskeletal pain and deterioration.** Back and neck pain are perhaps the most common and noticeable effects of spending our days sitting down. All that sitting also makes our muscles and bones weaker, meaning that, not only does getting active feel harder, but we're more prone to injury when we do.

This is by no means a complete list, and of course, it doesn't include the health effects of being overweight—and sitting's effects on your metabolism will definitely make weight loss more difficult. Research has popped up over the years linking "fidgety" or "hyperactive" traits with lower body weight. These studies always seemed a little odd, because the subjects were never moving enough to burn a ton of calories, but knowing what I know now, it makes perfect sense. I am sure you know someone like this in your life, who never seems to sit down or be still. Always on the move, cleaning, straightening, walking and talking, running errands. They are keeping their systems moving. Think of a car idling all day, engine running, versus one left parked in the garage except for a quick daily race around a track.

THE MOVING TARGET

I am asking you to add an extra 100 minutes of movement to your life every week. Let me be totally clear: I want 100 minutes *outside* of your exercise, and on top of whatever your current "baseline" is now. So even if you get forty-five minutes of exercise for a kickboxing class, you still need those ten to fifteen minutes of extra movement for this target. If you walk to work already, those minutes don't count toward your 100. But this target—like the target of 100 ounces of water—is one with a big payoff for relatively little effort. Adding just 100 minutes of movement to your week will make you feel noticeably better almost immediately, and as you'll see, getting more movement in your day has a pretty low barrier for entry; it is just a matter of creating the habit. You don't have to fight cravings or brave discomfort, and you don't need any equipment or special gear. I am a stickler for having comfortable shoes, because I hate it so much when my feet hurt, but that's about it. I'll talk more later about why I love using a wearable fitness tracker for this target, but if you are not a technology person, don't worry about it: this target was intentionally created using minutes instead of steps. Another reason I love adding movement is that it gets less "food drama" started for my clients than exercise does, while still having the benefit of increasing metabolism. Not only can exercise make people hungry, many struggle with feeling they have "earned" more food, or feel they need a food-related reward for their effort. It is a mind-set that has been established over time, and that mental habit can be hard to break. Adding movement does not seem to kick off that same mental process for my clients. Increasing movement will certainly burn more calories, but it doesn't trigger the old patterned thinking that makes clients feel the need to eat those calories back. Sparking metabolism without sparking cravings and mental baggage means progress is almost effortless.

So what does this target look like in practice? It's as simple as adding ten to fifteen minutes of walking to each day of the week. Take a twenty-minute walk after lunch every day during the workweek, or get up from your desk four times every workday and walk for five minutes with a friend. Take a thirty-minute walk after dinner, three nights a week. Do some gardening on the weekend, walk the dog, measure it and record it to make sure you are achieving your goal. This does not have to be difficult!

HIDDEN IN PLAIN SIGHT

The best part about this target is that you do not need to set aside a block of extra time like you would to go to a gym. You can fit it into your schedule as is, by finding "hidden time," time that is already accounted for but that you could spend moving. I swear, I can feel your skepticism as I write this, but it's true! Remember Mary's schedule, up above? Go ahead and take a look at it again. Mary was so discouraged by how little movement she was getting, and so sure there was no way she could fit more in. She and I sat down and systematically talked through her schedule, and guess what? We found places where she could get up and move, places that had been right in front of her. For example, her son's baseball games: naturally, she spent that time sitting on the bleachers. We got her walking around the field while watching the game instead. She did not need to find extra time for this; she was already at the field, but getting up from the bleachers had never occurred to her. Opportunities to move more are all around, but we are like horses with blinders on, plodding along the paths of our routines. The key is to create awareness of these opportunities and then use the habit loop to create a *new* routine.

One of the best examples of this is what happened when I was working with Joan. Joan is a bus driver—she loves the kids to death, but it is a hard job. She starts early and then is seated for most of the day. As we tried to figure out where she could fit movement in, I asked her to walk me through every hour, one by one. She was up and driving the bus at six, picking up kids all the way until a little after 9:30 AM, when they had all been delivered to school. At that point she pulled the bus around the side of the building, by the track, to wait for just over an hour before she began carting kids again. I stared at her for a minute. "You park the bus where?"

"Next to the track," she said.

"And what do you do for that hour, next to the track?"

"Wait on the bus." As the words left her mouth I saw the light bulb come on. She couldn't believe this option had been literally in front of her all along. For some reason we have a hard time identifying these opportunities for ourselves. I've had clients with full gyms in their basements tell me they can't work out because they don't want to leave the kids alone. I ask why they don't head down for a quick walk on the treadmill while the kids nap, and they look at me like I am a genius.

> **D-ficiency.** It is estimated that 85 percent of the American population is deficient in vitamin D. Lack of this vitamin will make you feel tired and sluggish. And not only does vitamin D boost metabolism, it is a potent anti-inflammatory agent that may play a role in preventing cancer and heart disease. So get outside every chance you get!

To return to Mary, we realized that her office was less than a mile from the train, and that it took her just as long to wait for the subway and get to her office that way as it would to walk the route instead. This added almost two miles of walking—an extra 2,000 steps each way—to her day. The walk gave her some much-needed stress relief at both the beginning and end of her workday. It got her a little fresh air and vitamin D she'd missed by riding the subway underground. The new routine was hard for Mary to settle into at first, and it made her uncomfortable for a few days while she got used to walking while carrying her work bag (and figured out which shoes worked best), but soon she couldn't imagine why she had ever taken the subway. (She saved a bunch of money, too!)

Take off the blinders and open your eyes to all the moments in your life that you spend sitting, and then systematically add movement. Treat it like a game: What can you do within your already-existing schedule to move more? Use the Hourly Movement Investigation worksheet below to go through your day, hour by hour. Could you fit in a walk first thing in the morning? Could you spend the half hour you devote to reading on your lunch break walking and listening to an audiobook instead?

MOVEMENT INVESTIGATION WORKSHEET

HOUR OF DAY	WHAT ARE YOU USUALLY DOING DURING THIS HOUR?	ACTIVE/ NOT ACTIVE?
5:00		
6:00		
7:00		
8:00		
9:00		
10:00		
11:00		
12:00		
1:00		
2:00		
3:00		
4:00		
5:00		
6:00		
7:00		
8:00		
9:00		
10:00		
11:00		

WEARABLES—NOT JUST ABOUT STEPS

I am a huge fan of wearable technology. I was part of the team that tested and developed the first wearable trackers at Weight Watchers, and secretly supplied Jennifer Hudson with one during her weight-loss journey. Jennifer fell in love with her device. She even tucked it in her waistband while onstage because she wanted "credit" for all her movement during performances! After leaving Weight Watchers, I consulted at several wearable device companies, and it was thrilling to see the technology evolve. Traditional pedometers used a pendulum-like measurement device, which only captured a forward, swinging motion, but the new wearable trackers were fitted with an accelerometer that could sense and quantify much more complex types of movement. Suddenly they could measure things like weight lifting and yoga. Over the years they've added more and more measurements—the ability to track sleep, heart rate, and even stress levels—and there are endless styles, from those you can carry discreetly in a pocket to bejeweled, flaunt-worthy bracelets.

> **Step Up.** Fitbits and similar fitness trackers are everywhere these days—many of them sitting in drawers. It's estimated that over 50 percent of the wearables purchased are never set up. I actually get this. I think people see the device as another "magic bullet" for fitness or weight loss. They buy it filled with hope and a sense of possibility, but taking it out of the box and setting it up signifies a commitment they aren't really ready to make. It's true, there are no magic bullets. But a wearable device can be a powerful tool as you set out to move more.

Like I said, this target is measured in minutes, not steps, specifically to make it as easy as possible—walking is free, and I'm betting you know how to tell time. However, I really recommend giving a wearable fitness tracker a try. One reason I like them so much is that the device itself ends up serving as a trigger. You see the band on your wrist and it reminds you to get moving. I love that often the devices themselves or connected apps can be set up like alarms to remind you to walk more. It can be helpful and motivating to have another way to quantify just how much extra movement your new habits are generating. These devices and their applications do a great job of engaging your naturally competitive nature: they prompt you to set goals, they display progress in visually interesting graphs. When you get a high number, you feel like your activity has been acknowledged and validated; when you glance at the display and find that the number is lower than usual, you might change your behavior to catch up. I love the fact that most platforms let you set challenges with friends, using healthy competition to create an environment that supports your goals.

You don't need a fancy two-hundred-dollar device to reap most of these benefits: you can purchase a good old-fashioned pedometer for less than ten bucks. Honestly, this is what Jessica Simpson used as she was working to get moving again after her pregnancies. Jessica's amazing personal trainer, Harley Pasternak, knew that Jessica needed to recover from pregnancy slowly and that walking would be the easiest effective way to get weight off, so he gave pedometers to Jessica and all of her friends in our Weight Watchers group. Jessica is an overachiever with a competitive streak, and this simple device inspired and motivated her. Giving pedometers to her friends as well was brilliant—we created a friendly competition and had a great time sending emails around about who was winning our little "Step War." Suddenly, something daunting—getting back in shape post-baby—was fun. Involving friends and family will help you establish the habit. My kids both have Fitbits and *love* them. They compete with me and each other to see who can get the most steps in a day. Honestly, my kids love that *I* have a Fitbit because my desire to rack up steps means I'm more likely to join them in a Nerf basketball game instead of flopping down on the couch after work—otherwise I don't stand a chance of winning a step race against two active boys. (What can I say, I like to win!)

MOVING FORWARD

Remember Newton's Law? *A body at rest tends to stay at rest.* You will not simply "remember" to move more. You'll need to rely on our old friend the habit loop, investigating your day for opportunities and triggering movement at certain points until it becomes a habit. That will take time. Mary's habit of taking the subway was so deep that we had to trigger those walks with alarms on her phone at each end of the route at the approximate time she would need them. And remember her plan to walk around the field at her son's baseball games? She will not arrive at the game and automatically start looping the field. She's tired, and her instinct will be to head to her usual spot on the bleachers. Maybe she'll walk for a game or two, and then the next time she'll think, "I'll just sit for a minute first." Getting the habit established is crucial, and without a reminder she is dead in the water. She needs to set alarms, or ask a friend to walk with her, or maybe bring the dog along to get her up and moving. But once Mary's spent enough games walking around the field, *that* becomes her default behavior—and it happens faster than you think!

The habit of movement can be established quickly, but will take tending and protecting to sustain long term, as our lives and schedules change. I have experienced this firsthand: I began writing this book just after my kids got out of school for the summer. I wasn't tracking movement, but had tracked for a long time in the past and felt confident that I was still getting somewhere around my usual 20,000 steps a day. Little did I realize how much more sedentary I'd become due to this massive change in my work life and the loss of walks to and from school with

WORDS OF LIZDOM

Reinvestigate your levels of movement periodically. Seasonal changes and schedule changes can suck activity away unnoticed.

the kids—I entered into a weeklong steps challenge with some members of my boot camp to find I had lost over 10,000 steps a day! Maybe it should have been obvious, now that the majority of my day was spent writing at my computer, but I was still making an effort to be active and so I was totally shocked. It forced me to trigger new routines, like setting an alarm to go off every hour, reminding me to get up and move. I began taking any and all phone calls standing up, walking around wearing a headset. I found ways within my new schedule to get my steps back where I needed them for my own weight maintenance. As I've said time and again, this journey does not end. Even those of us "in the business" must put effort into maintaining our healthy lifestyles.

The target of 100 minutes is meant to be a starting point. My ultimate goal for you isn't about a number of minutes. You can hit your target by taking three roughly half-hour walks a week and sitting perfectly still the rest of the time (except for exercise), but my hope is that, as you see the impact of more movement in your life, you will begin to add it everywhere. Happily, we have another piece of Newton's first law working in our favor: A body in motion tends to *stay* in motion. If you can begin to trigger yourself to move, I've found that more movement will naturally spring from that effort. As long as you're up, you'll find yourself puttering around the house, carrying laundry upstairs, taking a watering can outside to the garden. Your fifteen-minute walks will stretch to twenty and then twenty-five; friends from your office will ask to join you for your lunchtime stroll, or your kids will tag along on a walk to the store. Before you know it you will have created a new culture of movement in your life, one that sustains itself.

HABIT LIBRARY

1. Stand up and walk while on the phone.
2. Get a standing desk or elevate your computer so that you can stand periodically throughout your workday.
3. Set alarms to remind you to stand every thirty minutes.
4. Add walking to your commute—if you drive, park your car farther from work.
5. Walk the dog!
6. Walk the kids to school, to the bus stop, or to a park.
7. Ask a friend to join you for a walk.
8. Get a wearable device, pedometer, or an app that counts steps on your phone.
9. Buy a comfortable pair of shoes.
10. Walk after dinner for fifteen minutes.
11. Stand during commercial breaks while watching TV. Or, if you are streaming a show (or watching more than one), go for a ten-minute walk before each episode.
12. Play outside with the kids (or a dog).
13. Look up local hiking paths and plan a weekend hike.
14. Think through which errands (Bank? Post office?) you could perform by walking instead of driving.
15. Change up your route—walk a different part of your neighborhood.
16. Attach walking to an already-existing habit—like right after your morning coffee.
17. Use a walking-route app on your phone to measure your distance and time.
18. Add one extra minute of walking every day for seven days.
19. Make a plan for bad weather days: visit a mall, get an indoor walking DVD, or walk the stairs in your house or at work.
20. Join a local walking group.
21. Sign up to walk a 5K.
22. Make a list of the benefits you notice and how you feel after you walk.
23. Get off public transportation one stop early and walk the rest of the way.
24. Leave a note on the couch that reminds you to stay off of it!
25. Establish nonfood rewards for achieving your movement goals.

TARGETS
5 AND 6

STRESS
AND SLEEP

Chapter 8

STRESS LESS

You can do everything "right" in your weight-loss program and have all your work undone by something you may have never even considered: stress. Most weight-loss programs talk about just two things: food and exercise (and mostly food). The industry in general continues to be splintered, offering either demanding and rigid food plans or strenuous exercise regimens as stand-alone fixes. Food and exercise are important, and focusing on those areas alone can give you short-term success, but without addressing the way you deal with stress and other emotions—your long-standing habits and physical responses— you will eventually return to a higher weight. I know this isn't what you want to hear, but no one has long-term success managing weight without addressing *all* of the factors that affect it, and that includes stress and sleep, habit and environment, hydration and movement. If weight loss were as straightforward as simplistic marketing messages would have you believe, don't you think we would be making more headway? This realization can seem overwhelming. It was nice to believe we could pick up any diet plan and do it for some prescribed period of time and completely transform ourselves for good. I wanted that to be true myself, but I also know from experience that it's not.

As I've mentioned, I was a pro at fad diets when I was younger, taking off thirty pounds or so at a time. Inevitably, I'd watch those pounds return—but I kept trying, sure the perfect program was out there. I was a good student, reading the latest diet book and following the rules like commandments. In 2001, I was following a program that prescribed eating just enough protein to fill the palm of your hand and an accompanying vegetable portion of the same size. There was a list of forbidden foods and I avoided them like the plague. The plan prescribed six mini-meals spaced exactly a certain number of hours apart, so I lived by the clock. Believe it or not, it worked! I took the weight off and swore I would *never* go back. (Sound familiar?) The week after I reached my goal, the country was devastated by 9/11.

I lived and worked in New York City, and the stress levels I felt in the wake of the attacks were like nothing I had experienced before. I found myself panicking on every subway trip, my heart pounding with fear. We didn't know whether there would be more attacks, and it felt like the whole city was on hyperalert. Sleep was hard to come by. I went from obsessing about my weight to just being glad to be alive, and turned to food and alcohol in an endless stream of alternately celebratory and grief-stricken blowouts. The weight came rushing back, plus more. None of the things I had been doing to control my weight were even *remotely* a natural fit for my life, so when faced with large amounts of stress, they gave way completely. I got no comfort from my six mini-meals, and I reached instinctively for the old behaviors and habits I'd comforted myself with in the past.

This may seem like an extreme example, but stressful events, be they truly horrific or the more typical stresses of daily life, can be a tipping point. Stress can take you from totally dedicated to a "new" healthy lifestyle to not caring at all. Stress has likely acted as your "release valve" at some point, your reason for ditching a diet. It feels like the right thing to do in the moment, but it is a habit that keeps us from success. I'd hear a voice in my head—in response to work pressure, sick kids, family drama—saying, "With everything going on right now I just *can't* stick with this plan," and off I went. For a long, long time, that was my habit when faced with stress. All these years later, I know it was more than a psychological response, it was a physiological one as well. It was a reaction to a powerful chemical and hormonal process taking place deep in my brain and throughout my body. But over time we can learn to defuse stress—the everyday and even the epic. We can reduce the stress in our lives and develop the habit of managing it.

WORRIED SICK

Stress is a silent enemy that for many is a constant, low-level presence, always there, draining us while escaping our notice, a threat we don't deal with until it reaches a critical level and becomes suddenly urgent. Stress is built into our environment, and we've come to accept it as "normal," as if we have no choice in the matter. We have demanding jobs that offer vacation days we are too busy to take. Phones that make us reachable at all hours and let us bring the office with us wherever we go. A constant barrage of information via a twenty-four-hour news cycle and alarmist internet headlines fighting for our clicks. Increasingly burdensome ideas of what constitutes "good parenting" and social-media–driven expectations that our lives be Instagram-worthy at all times. Crowded schedules and long commutes, rising debt and financial worries. What's worse, we've developed habits and behaviors—our dependence on smartphones, our lack of stress-busting exercise—that make it worse.

What happens in your body when you are stressed? And how does it affect your weight? Allow me to totally oversimplify a very complex system: stress builds a wall against weight loss. Your body has a highly effective stress response system that kicks in when you sense danger, and it works to keep you safe. It begins in the brain: Imagine that you are walking in the forest and see a mountain lion. Your brain sends a lightning-fast signal and releases adrenaline into the bloodstream. Adrenaline is the hormone responsible for making you run faster than you ever knew you could, the hormone that gives people the superhuman strength to lift a car off a loved one. This reaction is known as the "fight-or-flight" response: your heart rate increases, breathing quickens, muscles tighten, and blood pressure rises. You're ready to act—this is how you protect yourself.

Now, you're probably not running into many mountain lions in your daily life, but unfortunately this response has not evolved along with our environment. Small things like being late for an important work meeting or realizing you've missed a bill payment can act as the catalyst to get the process started. One of the most important features of our body's stress response is its speed and the fact that it can be triggered without us being aware of it—the body doesn't wait around for the mountain lion to pounce, it springs into action as soon as it hears the crack of twigs in the underbrush. All day, as we race through our hectic schedules and worry about our to-do lists, we are triggering this response. It may never spike as high as it would in a truly dire situation, but it revs again and again in a series of smaller peaks.

Here's where weight comes in: To power your run away from danger, your body goes in and grabs a bit of fat from your fat stores and releases sugar into the bloodstream. It grabs only a tiny amount but assumes it will be needing more—the stress response, you see, is metabolically "expensive"—so after this the body releases the hormone cortisol to ensure it gets the extra energy it will need to survive the stress. Cortisol keeps blood sugar up and starts signaling the body to replenish your fuel supply. It tells you to gravitate toward food to replace the fat and sugar your body fears it will be losing. Each stress event is a small appetite booster—and it won't make you crave carrots. Nope, you're more likely to reach for cookies or mac and cheese (there's a reason they're called "comfort foods"). You are not doing anything wrong! This is a normal and necessary response in an emergency, but in today's world it's simply overkill.

Over time, we build habits around stress. We are pushed to high-fat, sugary, salty foods by our bodies, repeatedly, until it becomes our habit to eat when stressed. Now that you know how habits work, you can understand how this one is reinforced over time, as stress becomes the trigger and the consumption of fatty sugary foods releases dopamine as a reward.

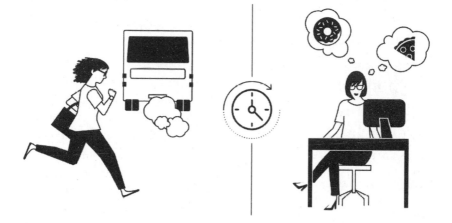

Depending on the long-term impact of whatever's stressing you out—and how you personally handle stress—it could take anywhere from half an hour to a couple of days to return to your resting state. Long-term exposure to high levels of cortisol has serious health risks, and it is crucial that our bodies have a chance to return to normal following a stressful event. Unfortunately, in today's high-stress culture, the stress response is activated so frequently that this often doesn't happen. You are living in that stress state most of the time, and your body is doing what it feels it must to survive. It is pumping that cortisol, increasing your appetite, building its fat stores. I don't think I have ever had a client who didn't cite "stress eating" as a problem. Many people report that they've found themselves eating almost on autopilot in response to stress. We have used food to soothe ourselves for so long, it is now a deeply ingrained behavior. You can imagine why your best-laid "diets" so often go awry.

Weight aside, stress is one of the most potently dangerous threats to our health. We *should* think of stress relief as vital, lifesaving medicine. But

Remember, your body is smarter than you. You can follow any weight-loss plan you like, but until you address your level of stress and your responses to it, your body will fight you the whole way—and it will usually win.

for some reason, even when clients know stress increases their risks for hundreds of diseases, they aren't motivated to fight it until they realize it affects weight loss—and most have no idea it does. Recently, one of my new boot camp clients told me she'd been working tirelessly to lose weight by cutting calories and yet was at a standstill. She'd become so upset about this that she even visited her doctor to have her thyroid checked. When tests showed her thyroid was functioning well, her doctor immediately began asking about her stress levels and sleep patterns. She had recently experienced a loss in her family and was sad and stressed and not sleeping well. Her doctor's prescriptions were stress-reducing exercises and breathing techniques. I was thrilled to hear that this is becoming a more common part of the conversation around weight, and my client was excited when our group covered stress reduction—she started using a meditation app on her phone and is feeling much better (and shedding pounds again), having added yoga and some journaling during the week to relax.

IDENTIFYING STRESS

As I started to work with clients on stress reduction, I was surprised to find that many didn't really know what stress "feels" like. They were experiencing some (or many) symptoms of stress, but were so used to constant, low-level stress that they didn't identify these as "symptoms" of anything—it was just the way they were used to feeling. They often weren't able to identify when stress began to build or what kicked it off. Sure, they could recognize a full-blown anxiety attack, but they usually didn't notice their stress levels rising until those levels were high enough to be really upsetting. By then, the stress response is already running at full throttle, spilling adrenaline, sugar, and cortisol into the bloodstream. We need to disrupt the process early, before it takes over, but we can't stop what we don't notice.

It is vitally important that we learn to notice when stress begins and how it feels: Stress signals, much like hunger signals, can be very individual, but with practice, you can become acutely aware of your own stress triggers and symptoms. Here is a chart that gives you an idea of the wide variety of ways in which stress can manifest:

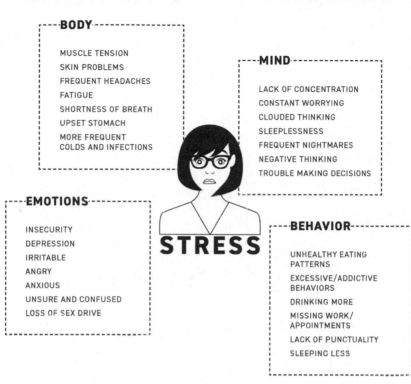

BODY

MUSCLE TENSION
SKIN PROBLEMS
FREQUENT HEADACHES
FATIGUE
SHORTNESS OF BREATH
UPSET STOMACH
MORE FREQUENT
COLDS AND INFECTIONS

MIND

LACK OF CONCENTRATION
CONSTANT WORRYING
CLOUDED THINKING
SLEEPLESSNESS
FREQUENT NIGHTMARES
NEGATIVE THINKING
TROUBLE MAKING DECISIONS

EMOTIONS

INSECURITY
DEPRESSION
IRRITABLE
ANGRY
ANXIOUS
UNSURE AND CONFUSED
LOSS OF SEX DRIVE

STRESS

BEHAVIOR

UNHEALTHY EATING
PATTERNS
EXCESSIVE/ADDICTIVE
BEHAVIORS
DRINKING MORE
MISSING WORK/
APPOINTMENTS
LACK OF PUNCTUALITY
SLEEPING LESS

Now, take a minute to think about your own responses to stress.

WHAT STRESS FEELS LIKE FOR ME

Body:

_____

Emotions:

_____

Behavior:

_____

Brain:

_____

What are the most stressful things in your life right now?

_____

What do you know, for a fact, reduces your stress levels?

_____

What new stress reliever are you willing to try?

_____

TARGETING STRESS

This target asks you to aim for 100 minutes of stress relief each week. What does that look like? The answer may be completely different for each of us. I return you to the idea that this is *your* program. You may decide that one hour-long yoga class alongside two twenty-minute walks at lunch is your weekly formula. I choose to do five twenty-minute meditation sessions each week. (I like that I have two days off to work with so that my de-stressing minutes don't stress me out!) Some people feel most refreshed by restful, contemplative activities, while others find they need to do something active that gets them "out of their own head." Mindfulness exercises can fit either description, depending on the specific type you do, as can yoga.

I love meditation, but it took some time to get comfortable with it and find a type that worked for me. I have clients who love coloring or knitting for stress relief, and others who run, or read, or garden, or write in a journal. One woman I know swears by putting on loud music and having a solo dance party (or a dance party with the kids), and another bakes bread and elaborate cakes. I find that my dog, Angus, is just about the best form of stress relief I have. He seems to appear right at the moment I need him most, to take me on a walk or just to snuggle. I try to take advantage of this every time I can, whether by getting outside for a walk or simply taking a few moments to get down on the ground and let him make me smile a little. Think outside the box when it comes to stress-relieving activities—almost anything you enjoy can count if you find it leaves you feeling relaxed.

Here are some of the most common:

- Breathing exercises
- Meditation
- Spending time with a pet or animals
- Listening to music
- Yoga
- Coloring
- Knitting
- Calling a friend
- Positive visualization
- Taking a walk
- Journaling
- Making a "gratitude list"
- Spending time outdoors
- Taking a bath
- Getting a massage

Banish Guilt. I get pushback on this target—especially from women, and double especially from women with kids—for one big reason: guilt. Taking half an hour to color or soak in a leisurely bath feels frivolous. It's easy to say you'll relax later, when no one else needs anything from you and every item on your to-do list is checked off, but guess what? *That moment will never come.* There will always be something else you could be doing. Making time for yourself isn't selfish, it's smart. So if you find yourself feeling guilty, push back against those thoughts! Remind yourself that nothing on your to-do list is more important than your health, and that time spent "unwinding" is every bit as vital to your health as eating well or exercising.

I am asking you to aim for 100 minutes of stress relief *on top* of your exercise and movement minutes. Exercise is an amazing stress reliever: it produces endorphins—chemicals in the brain that act as natural painkillers—and improves sleep, which in turn reduces stress. If your stress relief activity of choice is exercise or taking a walk, that's great . . . but those minutes only count for one target at a time. Keeping your minutes separate underscores your commitment to focusing on each and every one of the six targets. Ultimately, trying to find ways to "cheat" the program makes no sense: after all, this is your program. If you feel overwhelmed, how about making time this week for just one ten-minute session of whatever feels like a de-stressor to you. Then, add ten more minutes next week, and so on. Don't let stress relief—or any of the targets—become a source of stress!

HOW MEDITATION BECAME MY TOP WEIGHT-LOSS TIP

People have been asking me for weight-loss tips for fifteen years. And over the years, my "top weight-loss tip" has changed several times. Years ago it was "track your food," then it was "get support," and later "separate movement from exercise." As times have changed, our challenges have evolved. We have battled increasingly processed foods, become ever more sedentary, and added endless distractions to our day through technology. In a recent interview, asked what my number one weight-loss tip would be, I surprised myself with my own answer—because it had nothing to do with food or exercise. Today, I believe the number one thing you can do to see more progress toward your weight-loss goal is to begin a meditation practice.

Why? Our current environment of ever-present distraction and temptation is destroying our ability to stay focused on long-term goals, especially when it comes to weight loss. Clients come to me shocked by recent rapid weight gain because they don't "feel like" they are eating much more than they used to. They find themselves eating when they are not even hungry, and more and more report feeling like food is controlling them. I am not surprised they have gained weight without even realizing it, because their behavior has become mindless, much of it driven by outside forces.

Most of us have enough to eat, and these days we are increasingly driven by the pleasure we derive from food rather than by any actual need. Scientists refer to this as "hedonic hunger." Factors like stress drive us to seek out food we don't need and then reward us with a burst of dopamine, and stoking the fires of excess consumption are the continual food cues blasted at us throughout the day. Remember, humans respond to food when we are exposed to it—when we see images of it, smell it, or even talk about it—and from the moment we wake up, we are drowning in these triggers, through ads on our smartphones, billboards along the drive to work, pop-ups on our computers, and commercials on TV. Each is a subtle marketing message urging you away from your good intentions, and these messages are running all day in the background of every part of our lives.

Meditation is, hands down, the most effective tool I have found for helping clients learn to cut through the eternal background noise and find calm and clarity. It gives them the awareness they need of their thoughts and actions, the ability to focus their attention throughout the day. By teaching us to be more mindful, meditation gives us some of our control back.

You don't have to take my word for it, either. The benefits of meditation, especially mindfulness meditation, are one of the few things scientists seem to agree upon! I'm not sure I have ever seen anything in the wellness world with so much research backing it up. Meditation has been shown in study after study to have a positive impact on just about anything we can think of, from mood and mental performance to risks of cancer and heart disease. It is proven to improve our ability to focus and overcome distractions, to help us manage stress, to reduce anxiety and depression, to improve sleep, and boost the immune system.

Another reason I love to prescribe meditation is that you can do it anywhere. You don't need any equipment at all, just a quiet spot to close your eyes. Start slowly, with five or ten minutes, and be patient! I promise the benefits are worth it. Many people think you have to be able to "clear your mind of all thoughts" to meditate, but that isn't true—when thoughts pop into your head, you simply notice them and then return your focus to your breath or your body, over and over. Meditation is about learning to be fully in the present, and it is a skill like any other, one you can *absolutely* master with a little practice. There are a ton of great apps and podcasts about meditation to explore. Try out different types until you find what works for you—there is walking meditation, mantra meditation, guided meditation, and many others—and experiment with different times of day as well. I find it especially effective to meditate right after a workout. Your body is alive and awake and your awareness of it is heightened, and at the same time you're maybe even a little bit tired, so you can relax pretty quickly. I have a client in my gym every day by around 5:30 AM. At the end of each session, I take them through a quick guided meditation. I play music and talk through

STRESS RELIEF ON THE RUN

Stress can pop up unexpectedly, and we don't always have the luxury of our favorite de-stressing activity when it does. Build a toolbox of simple, do-anywhere strategies for stopping stress in its tracks. Here are five to get you started:

- **Meditation or breathing exercises.** Download a meditation app on your phone and carry a pair of earphones in your bag for spur-of-the-moment serenity. Or, do some relaxation breathing—focus on breathing deeply into your abdomen, and breathe so that the exhale is longer than the inhale (for example by breathing in for a count of four and then out for a count of eight).

- **Essential oils.** Essential oils like lavender can have an immediate calming effect. Find one that works for you, and carry it in your purse or on a piece of paper slipped into your wallet.

- **Mantras or quotes.** It may sound cheesy, but having a calming affirmation to turn to can work wonders in a time of crisis. Pick something easy to remember and meaningful to you—it can be as simple as "I am strong"—and when you feel stress mounting, repeat it to yourself.

- **Pressure points.** Look online and familiarize yourself with pressure points that relieve anxiety—one is on the inside of the wrist, about three fingers down from the crease where the wrist meets your hand. These can be a discreet way to halt the stress response.

- **Chocolate.** Dark chocolate contains anandamide, a substance that blocks pain and gives us a quick shot of feel-good chemicals. Carry an individually wrapped square in your bag for an emergency!

some body scanning and visualizations to set them up for a day of calm and focus. You can easily do the same thing for yourself using a meditation app or by searching YouTube for "guided meditation." Doing meditation at the end of an exercise session is not only effective, it is a great way to "piggyback" one habit onto another. Once you have established the exercise habit, it can act as your trigger for the habit of meditation!

The results will be subtle at first. You will likely notice that you are more confident, not as anxious, and are ultimately more in control of your eating and food choices. Long term, developing a meditation practice will serve you well through every season of your life, helping you handle whatever challenges are thrown your way.

BEYOND STRESS RELIEF—BREAKING THE STRESS HABIT

This target is not just about creating a new habit—taking time for stress relief—it is about breaking an old habit as well: the habit of stress. Stress, believe it or not, is often a habit, something we've built into our lives and reinforced. Of course, plenty of stress is due to forces beyond our control, but I guarantee that you have stress-creating habits adding to the problem. Remember the Behavior Modification Worksheet we did way back in Chapter One? Take a look at the three major obstacles you identified as standing in your way. I'll bet most of these can be traced back to behaviors that are creating and exacerbating stress. Let me give you an example:

My sister Catherine came to one of my workshops, where we walked through that Behavior Modification Worksheet as a group. She realized that she has a real problem saying no in her life. As we discussed it further, it became obvious that her habit of saying yes to everything was leaving her with a packed schedule filled with projects and events that she often had no desire—or time—to participate in. That, in turn, was creating stress, resentment, and even some residual anger that resulted in Catherine feeling a "need" to eat something that gave her an escape or something to look forward to. Sometimes she was so overscheduled that it was simply impossible to prepare a meal, and she was forced to grab something on the go—usually not until she was so ravenous that she had no hope of making a rational food decision. (Letting yourself get overhungry all but guarantees your good intentions will be shouted down by your appetite.)

This workshop was an "aha" moment for my sister. She realized that she needed practice saying no, and we decided that she would find a way to say no to something at least three times in the next week, even rehearsing her polite refusals in front of a mirror. She would also look through her schedule for at least two things that she could eliminate from her workload or calendar once her current commitment to them was finished. This is a perfect example of how misguided it is to focus only on food when you're trying to lose weight. Flexing that "no" muscle was difficult for my sister, but imagine if she'd just gone on a "diet," *without* addressing the underlying habit that was driving her poor eating choices. She might have gotten some weight off, but at some point, overscheduling and all of the emotions that it creates would drive her back to comforting herself with food, and the weight would return. Then, the next time, she would have the added burden of her past "failure" undermining her confidence. On the other hand, if she could get her schedule under control and find a way to release some stress through exercise, meditation, or rest, she would have the time and the focus to make food decisions driven by her goals, not by her emotions and the demands of her body's stress response. Until you get your stress under control, it will continue to control you.

Another of my clients, Stacey, is one of my favorite stress success stories. Stacey is funny and smart—she never fails to make me laugh, and no matter the topic, she always has a fresh perspective I've never considered. Stacey was also famous for being late. Everyone in her life knew this about her; it had become a part of her persona. It was also a habit that created an incredible amount of stress. Stacey is hardly unique—many clients report that one of their largest stressors is the feeling of "always running behind." This is partly why two of the most common things I work on with clients are their morning and evening routines. With Stacey, we focused first on her mornings, because they were such a mess that the situation was actually beginning to affect her work life. She was waking up late, getting sidetracked by the TV and computer while she drank her coffee, then—noticing the time—she'd end up skipping breakfast and racing to get ready, ultimately arriving at the office later than she should. She had recently been promoted and was managing several new employees. Her frantic mornings got her cortisol levels on the rise, and gave her little time to prep for the day ahead, and walking in late was making her self-conscious. She arrived at work feeling guilty and unprepared. In short, she was starting each day with a giant stress bomb.

We tackled Stacey's morning piece by piece. Many people—Stacey included—use a phone as their alarm clock and press snooze several times before getting out of bed, so they can "sleep" as long as possible. There are two separate problems here: First, it is horribly stressful to use the snooze button. Don't try to tell me that you are deeply refreshed by those seven-minute siestas. Either you drift off, only to be startled awake again almost immediately, or you lie there anxiously waiting for the alarm, thinking about the day ahead while you load your system with cortisol. You can make your mornings less stressful simply by setting an alarm clock all the way across the room and forcing yourself on your feet right away, before your thoughts have a chance to start racing—and before you snooze yourself late. The second problem is using your phone as an alarm clock—if you do this, I would bet money that the first thing you do after that alarm goes off is check your email or social media. This creates stress and anxiety right away, and sets you up for distraction and, you guessed it, starting the day behind schedule. I had Stacey buy a real alarm clock and get up just thirty minutes earlier. We also eliminated all screens in the morning: She would no longer watch TV or open her computer while she drank her coffee, but instead spent that time relaxing—looking out the window and cuddling with her sweet dog. Stacey had thought she was getting ahead by glancing at her email first thing in the morning and trying to get some work done before she hit the office. In fact, it was creating stress, making her late, and—because she was in a hurry and juggling her other morning tasks—she was usually only half focused anyway. Her new routine eliminated anxiety and helped her avoid getting sidetracked. By waking up earlier and leaving on time, she could walk, further reducing stress (when she was late, she'd been taking cabs and fretting about the money during the ride). Stacey now had time to grab her favorite healthy breakfast on her walk to the office, getting in early to look at email and prepare for the day's meetings with a clear mind and no distractions.

Starting mornings off on the right foot created the momentum she needed to make better decisions all day. Just by working on her lateness we moved mountains: Because she felt better all day, she had the energy to get to the gym after work. Going to the gym made her feel virtuous and inspired her to eat healthier dinners. Eating right and getting some exercise improved her sleep, making it easier to get up on time in the morning, and so on. Soon Stacey's career was thriving and her weight was on the way down. When you unravel the habits that are standing in your way, the rest begins to fall in place.

Dissect your routines and find the places where your actions are creating stress. Face them with no emotion: these are not moral failings. Attack them one at a time with surgical precision, using your habit-formation tools to replace them with new routines. In order to break Stacey's old morning habits and create new ones, we had to put sticky notes all over her house. We placed one on the TV reminding her to leave it off, one on her closed laptop reminding her not to open it. These "triggers" reminded her of her new routine. Ask for help if you can't see a way out of a habit, and don't be upset when a little relapse happens. Practice, not perfection!

WEIGHT SHOULDN'T BE STRESSFUL— HOW GAMIFICATION WORKS

So, we've learned that stress will stall your weight loss, which presents us with an interesting additional problem: Weight loss, itself, can be stressful. Think about the way most diet and weight-loss systems are set up. We've talked about this before—it is expected that you will sign up for their program or read their book and immediately upend your entire life. You are supposed to stop things, start things, say no to pleasure and yes to dozens of new to-do-list items. New foods, new rules, new exercises, new everything— all at once. Just thinking about it stresses me out! Target 100 tries to take the stress out of weight loss as much as possible. We've chosen a few habits to focus on, one at a time, waiting until we are ready to layer on something new. But small changes are still changes, and any weight-loss attempt, no matter how reasonable, requires you to stand by your decision to do things a new way while the world pushes in the opposite direction. Stress is all but unavoidable.

Imagine that you've settled into your new weight-loss program. You're past the initial "figuring it all out" stage—you've built new routines and are seeing results. Now you have a big event coming up, a wedding weekend with friends from school, and you begin to worry. You perceive it as a threat. What will your food options be? Will you be tempted to overeat or drink too much? Will there be social pressure? How will you handle it all? And so I am going to introduce you to one last stress-busting strategy: "gamification."

Take the example above. This kind of stress is exactly what I want my clients to avoid, so instead we look at that event as a game. We make it fun! We come up with ways to earn "points." We look at who our allies are, where the dangers lie, and how to avoid them. We laugh about it as we prepare for it. With so much stress built into our everyday lives, the last thing we need is to add to it by fretting over every new challenge. "Gamifying" reduces stress by changing the stories we tell ourselves about the difficulties we face, turning them into adventures.

You can take this same approach to your weight-loss effort as a whole. If we look at weight loss as a game, rather than a punishment, how might that change our feelings about it? Research is proving that gaming puts us into an open, problem-solving frame of mind and increases motivation. The same kids who get discouraged and want to give up as soon as their math homework gets difficult will work tirelessly at a complicated construction project in Minecraft that asks them to use the very same skills. When we play games, it stokes the parts of us that are optimistic, creative, focused, and resilient. We're more excited to work hard, and we're less afraid of failure.

I am ending this chapter with a worksheet you can use to reframe your weight-loss project. Perspective is everything. Losing weight is often fraught with the stress of the new and unknown, self-doubt born of past failures, and shame over having gained weight in the first place. It is a consequence, a burden, a penance—anything but fun. But try thinking of it as a secret mission, an adventure you've chosen, and your focus shifts to strategy. One at a time you work to master new levels. In the game of weight loss your enemies can be people, situations, even times of day, and allies and tools are everywhere. Will it be a new recipe, a friend, a meditation app, or a changed routine that catapults you past your next obstacle? In previous attempts, things like stress and lack of sleep worked stealthily against you, driving your choices and ultimately pushing you back to old behaviors. Once you identify them you can fight them off, enjoy finding ways to outwit them, and begin to have (stress-free) success that you never knew was possible.

WEIGHT LOSS AS A GAME

My Super-Secret Mission (describe your goals and what it will mean to complete your mission):

_____

_____

_____

The top three tools I have at my disposal:

1. _____

2. _____

3. _____

My top three allies:

1. _____

2. _____

3. _____

The top three enemies attempting to take me down (people, boredom, stress, emotional eating, work, schedule):

1. _____

2. _____

3. _____

My immediate plan of attack (for the next twenty-four hours) to ward off my enemies and move forward:

_____

_____

HABIT LIBRARY

1. Download a meditation app.
2. Practice deep breathing.
3. Stop using the snooze button.
4. Stop checking email once you are finished with work for the evening.
5. Write in a journal.
6. Begin a coloring routine.
7. Take a ten-minute walk outside at the peak stress time of your day.
8. Experiment with essential oils.
9. Make yourself a stress-relief first-aid kit.
10. Try a yoga class.
11. Reduce caffeine.
12. Listen to soothing music.
13. Disable notifications or use the "Do Not Disturb" function on your phone or computer to reduce distractions.
14. Call a friend.
15. Designate a schedule for checking your email or social media, and put your phone on a charger the rest of the time.
16. Take a day off from work.
17. Flip through photos of happy times.
18. Take a mindful walk, noticing your surroundings.
19. Make a gratitude list.
20. Spend time with an animal.
21. Have a piece of chocolate.
22. Read a book or watch a movie that makes you laugh.
23. Get a massage.
24. Play a game.
25. Take a bath.

Chapter 9

SLEEP YOUR WAY TO SUCCESS

I will admit that sleep was the last piece to fall into place as I began to think of developing my own program. After years of working in the mainstream weight-loss industry—which virtually ignores sleep—I had a lot to learn. I'd hear things from time to time about the impact of sleep on weight, but to be honest, I didn't really listen. I thought that sleep might affect weight loss for those with severe insomnia or sleep apnea, but not for average people with everyday sleep challenges. Then, a few years ago, I had the opportunity to meet and work alongside Dr. Michael Breus, America's "Sleep Doctor." We were serving as judges on Transformation Nation, Dr. Oz's yearlong health initiative, and spent several days together poring over the applications of those who hoped to win the grand prize. Sleep was one of the seven health indicators being considered, and the time I spent in that room alongside Dr. Breus and the other judges (among them Deepak Chopra, Dr. Oz, and even the deputy director of the CDC) was like a master class not only on sleep, but wellness as a whole. After meeting Dr. Breus, I read his books and found myself surprised and fascinated by the wide-ranging effects lack of sleep has on the body and brain. When you're not getting enough sleep, the resulting imbalance of hormones and decrease in overall performance is staggering. I began to address sleep with all of my clients, and I knew it would have to be one of the pillars of Target 100.

Sleep is a basic need, like nourishment and hydration. Unfortunately, what I hear from clients is that it has become a casualty of busy schedules, viewed as the most expendable piece in an increasingly demanding puzzle. Something has to give, right? People who would never think of starving themselves to save time see no problem with cutting back on sleep—it seems like the logical thing to do when you need extra hours in the day; we can't bend time, so we abuse our bodies. The pace of modern life has left us unable to catch up, and created an environment where "busyness" is a badge of honor. The result is the frazzled stay-at-home mom—whose husband works long hours to keep them financially afloat—responsible for three children and all of their activities, meals, and attendant tasks, who wakes in the night and finds herself unable to get back to sleep, running through the calendars and lists she keeps in her head. It's the working couple who are both gone from dawn to dusk, with long commutes and nonexistent work/life boundaries, checking email at 11 PM and pecking away at laptops in bed. The rapid rise of mobile technologies, unrealistic expectations, and demands for greater productivity and availability keep us running ragged. It's funny, when I interview new clients, we can often trace the beginnings of weight gain to times that included little sleep. Sometimes it is a loss in the family, sometimes it is a job change or the birth of a baby. Yet they rarely make the connection themselves, until I ask—it is the last place we look when we find ourselves gaining weight. We examine our food intake, our exercise routines, but our sleep habits never cross our minds.

THE PHYSIOLOGY OF SLEEP AND WEIGHT

I am not going to bore you with pages and pages about the mechanics of sleep and why it's important to your health. As with stress, the unfortunate truth is that knowing about the impact on health alone usually isn't enough to spur change. Instead, I am going to give you a layman's overview of how sleep impacts *weight*. Hopefully, this understanding will inspire you to do something about your sleep habits. The important word to recognize in that sentence is "habits." Your sleep is already habit driven—and luckily, by now you are an old pro at understanding and changing habits.

Sleep is the crucial time the body uses to recover after the day, to replenish, nourish, and detoxify itself. Forget juice "cleanses"—along with hydration, sleep is the most powerful detox there is. During sleep, the liver scrubs toxins from our system, the brain "washes" itself of waste, tissue is repaired throughout the body . . . and hormones are produced and regulated. When we don't get enough rest or that rest is fragmented, we disturb critical processes that support a healthy, balanced metabolism. Study after study reveals that those who sleep less than seven hours a night weigh more, gain more weight over time, and have a harder time losing weight. When we get less than seven hours of sleep, our levels of the appetite-boosting hormone ghrelin increase by about 15 percent while appetite-suppressing leptin *decreases* by the same amount. When you are short on sleep, you may notice

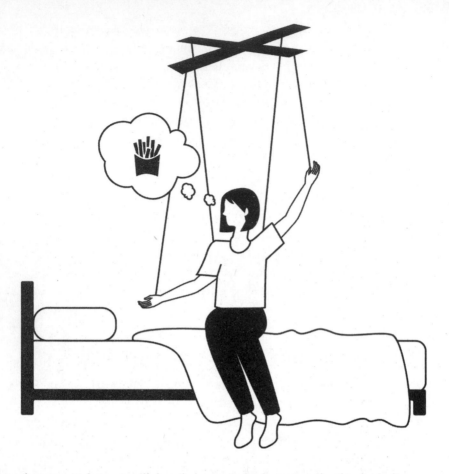

that you are hungrier all day; there are multiple reasons for this, including your desire for more energy and the mistaken idea that food will supply it, but it is this ghrelin/leptin imbalance that ultimately sends you heading for the vending machines. This imbalance is the genesis of that frustrating experience we've all had of wanting to stick to our healthy plans but feeling driven to seek out high-fat, salty, and sugary foods.

It may make you feel guilty, or as if something is wrong with you, but in fact something is right: This is a deep biological drive, an internal force that does not bow easily to "willpower" and does not care about your goals. Your body has one goal—to stay alive—and it is doing what it believes it needs to do based upon the way it is being treated. I'm going to repeat this, because it is just that important: **When you miss sleep, the hormone that tells you it's time to eat increases by 15 percent while the hormone that signals you to *stop* eating decreases by 15 percent.** That is a massive disadvantage you are battling. It's like starting a baseball game five runs down.

Another, potentially more serious problem is that it only takes about four days of sleep deprivation to throw off your body's response to insulin. Insulin is the hormone that tells your body that your blood sugar is high enough and signals it to store fat. Studies at the University of Chicago show that after just a few days of shortened sleep times, sensitivity to insulin drops by more than 30 percent. If your body stops responding to insulin, fat and sugar stay in the bloodstream, and the pancreas releases more and more insulin until your body finally gets the message. But cells can only store so much glucose and fat, and by this point, scrambling, your body starts storing the excess in organs like the liver. Not only does insulin resistance increase the likelihood of gaining weight, it is the driving factor behind metabolic syndrome and what eventually leads to the development of type 2 diabetes. In a frustrating cycle, high blood-sugar levels from sleep deprivation prompt the body to try to get rid of extra sugar via the kidneys, making it more likely you'll wake in the night to go to the bathroom . . . further disrupting your sleep.

Deprive your body of sleep and you could follow the exact same diet as a well-rested friend and make a fraction of the progress. Many times I've seen diet gurus or program leaders look skeptically at clients who claim to be "doing everything right" and yet seeing few results. They respond with disbelief or by suggesting the client further restrict calories, sending a clear message: one of shame, suggesting the client must be at fault. Many who work in the weight-loss world still refuse to believe there is more to the equation than food and exercise, calories in and calories out. When I have a client who comes to me crying about doing "everything right" and getting nowhere, I know something else is going on, and I've found the most common "something else" is sleep. I wish someone had told me this earlier. After my sons were born, I had sixty-five and fifty pounds to lose, respectively. People had promised me that breast-feeding and getting back to healthy eating habits would "melt" the weight right off. Instead, I jumped onto a weight-loss plan and watched as almost nothing happened until each of my sons began regularly sleeping through the night. In retrospect, I wish that, along with tracking my food and exercise as I worked to lose weight after they were born, I had also tracked my sleep. I'll bet that the plateaus I experienced would line up nicely with times when the boys were not sleeping well—and so neither was I.

A few final sobering sleep facts:

Fact: People who miss out on sleep are stimulating the same brain system that marijuana activates to create the "munchies." In a study, sleep-deprived participants could literally not resist tempting food placed in front of them—even though they had already eaten a full meal. Those who were well rested could give the snacks a pass.

Fact: Those who sleep less than six hours a night actually have shorter life expectancies. Staying up late and waking early may feel like it's netting you extra time, but it's not.

Fact: Studies have found that when dieters cut back on sleep over a fourteen-day period, the amount of weight they lost from fat dropped by 55 percent, even though their calorie intake stayed the same. They also felt hungrier and less satisfied after meals, and suffered from low energy.

TARGETING ZZZS

This target calls for you to add 100 minutes of extra sleep a week. (Yes. I just asked you to sleep more. Who knew you could lose weight by spending more time in bed?) You may have heard that we "naturally" sleep for just as long as our bodies need to. Not in this day and age. Our natural sleep rhythms are a mess. Our environment has left many of us chronically sleep deprived, and not only are we not getting enough sleep, the quality of the sleep we do get is often very low. Each "stage" of sleep has important functions, and many of us are missing out on the deep sleep we need, due to waking in the night.

The standard recommendation is to get anywhere between seven and nine hours of sleep per night, but I have found that almost everyone has a much more specific amount of sleep they need to function at their best. This is probably not surprising to you. Even in my own family there is a great variance: my oldest son has never needed nearly as much sleep as my younger son does. I need at least seven hours most nights and work hard to get them. (Now that I am aware of how sleep deprivation drives my hunger and weight, I am very serious about my sleep!) This is another area where you'll need to be a bit of a scientist whose subject is yourself. Uncover the right amount of sleep for you by keeping track of your sleep and how you feel the next day. If you are one of the rare people who is getting enough sleep, you can use this target to focus on the quality of that sleep instead of adding minutes—most of us, however, will need to do both. Once in a while, poor-quality sleep actually causes someone to sleep too much without ever being fully rested. As I dig in with my clients, I almost always find multiple sleep issues. Adding minutes will force you to address factors, like bedtime routines, that also impact the quality of your sleep. Looking for ways to improve the quality of your sleep will make it easier for you to fall asleep and stay that way, ultimately adding sleep minutes. Again, you will have to do some investigation into your own sleep patterns. Do you find that the sun wakes you too early? Are you too hot at night? Do you wake up frequently on nights when you drink alcohol? Are you unable to fall asleep due to anxiety over the day ahead?

Our sleep struggles are as individual as we are, but every one of us can benefit from better sleep, and there are endless ways to improve it. Sleep is one of those things we take for granted as "natural," but healthier sleep habits will not happen magically. They must be consciously tackled, triggered, and consistently tended, just like any others.

SLEEP SECRETS

Our biggest problem is that we treat sleep like it should happen at the snap of our fingers. Because it is supposed to be "natural," we also see it

---

SLEEP MEDICINE

I have seen an alarming uptick in the prescription of sleep aids and am always hoping to move clients away from them to behavioral sleep strategies that often work just as well. Many prescription sleep aids have dangerous side effects, from memory loss to drug dependence, and most of these drugs actually result in lower-quality sleep! Sure, they help you fall asleep or stay asleep, but the price is disordered sleep cycles that lead to hormonal imbalances, or grogginess the next day that we fight off with caffeine—which only makes it harder to sleep at night. It should be clear to you by now that losing weight is all about keeping our body's systems working in balance, and anything that throws that balance off will have consequences.

However, there are some natural sleep aids that I recommend to clients who need a little bit of help as they begin to work on their sleep routines. Of course, before starting any herbal supplements, check with your doctor to avoid possible interactions with other drugs you may be taking.

- **Melatonin.** A hormone produced in your brain that regulates your body's sleep rhythms, melatonin can be a gentle way to encourage your body to fall asleep.
- **Chamomile.** Drinking a cup of chamomile tea before bed is a sleep strategy that has been used for centuries. Chamomile is also proven to work as an anti-inflammatory, to soothe the stomach, and to reduce anxiety.
- Valerian. Made from valerian root, this herbal supplement may not only help you fall asleep faster, it can also calm anxiety and lower blood pressure.
- **Magnesium.** This mineral is my favorite. It helps relax your muscles, and it's great for those suffering from restless leg syndrome. It is also a major player in the functioning of the neurotransmitters that calm your central nervous system. It won't necessarily make you magically drift off to dreamland, but it can help calm your body and make getting to sleep easier. Many people don't get enough magnesium, either, because they don't eat a balanced diet (nuts and green leafy vegetables are good sources of magnesium), or because they take certain drugs for heartburn and acid reflux that interfere with its absorption. You can up the magnesium in your diet, take it in pill form, or look for magnesium tablets or electrolyte drinks.

as somewhat mysterious. We have sleep all wrong, thinking of it as both more simplistic and more complicated than it really is. Imagining it like an on/off switch we can't quite control, we lie down and wait for it to flip. For some reason, while we frequently complain to friends and colleagues about being tired or busy or "up late," we act like it can't be helped, as if waking four or five times a night is inevitable, suffering in silence until we get desperate enough to begin taking sleep aids—many of which have side effects that actually make the problem worse. Magazine articles are filled with "tips" on how to get better sleep, but those tips can't be implemented without relying on habit-formation science. There are myriad environmental changes to consider, from light and sound to temperature, what to wear and what bedding to use, devices to try and advice to absorb. We read the articles, but this seldom translates into action because we do not approach sleep with the methodical determination we would a problem at work or an unhealthy diet, and our sleep habits are deeply ingrained. Sleep is such a habit-driven activity that we continue doing what we know "works," even if it doesn't work very well! Clients come to me with *terrible* sleep habits: dozing with the television on, on couches, or spending half of their nights in their children's beds, just to name a few. These sleep routines have become habit, and they don't want to mess with the status quo and risk a night of sleeplessness as they adjust to something new, unaware that they are torpedoing their weight loss. But sleep isn't a mysterious on/off switch that flips, sleep is a *process*—one that most of us have never had proper training in. We need to wind down, relax, and prepare for sleep. It should be planned for and protected the way we would any of the other important activities in our lives, like work, meals, or exercise. Viewing sleep as a process is a difficult jump to make, but once you do, you'll see there is a logical place to begin your work on this target: with your morning and evening routines.

REVISITING ROUTINES

We've looked at morning and evening routines through the lenses of many other targets, from food to stress, but they are perhaps more crucial than ever when it comes to sleep. How much and how well you sleep are the direct result of these routines, and inevitably, I hear that clients have given them little thought. These critical moments of our day are haphazard and disorganized at best. I watch friends construct carefully considered bedtime routines for their children while completely ignoring their own. Why do we think this is less important for us? In fact, as we age, our systems are increasingly less resilient, making the renewing properties of sleep more vital than ever, while the pressures of adult life make the transition from stress to rest more difficult.

In the previous chapter, we talked about my client Stacey's morning routine, and how remaking that routine allowed her to defeat the chronic lateness that was setting her up for a day of stress and poor choices. It probably won't surprise you to hear that her evening routine was equally chaotic. Most nights Stacey was working on her laptop—while also watching TV—until right before bed.

Morning and evening are sacred times. Protect them by establishing routines that are both restful and rejuvenating. These routines are a cornerstone of your weight-loss success.

She often struggled with late-night snacking (driven by commercials on TV, banner ads on her computer, and being up for so many hours after dinner) and had trouble falling asleep, no doubt in part because of spikes in her blood sugar (and all that screen time—studies show that the light emitted by screens can disrupt your sleep all night long). Her lack of sleep contributed to her difficulty getting up in the morning, which of course contributed to her stress and feeling behind at work, which in turn made her more likely to stay up late working—you can see how all the targets, and sleep and stress in particular, are deeply intertwined.

We created a new nighttime routine for Stacey, one that would support the process of sleep. She set an alarm on her phone for 10 PM each night, alerting her to turn off her computer, turn lights down around the apartment, and begin her bedtime routine. She then spent the next thirty minutes brushing her teeth, getting into her PJs, and cleaning up a bit so she wouldn't wake to a mess. She also took a magnesium supplement (a natural sleep aid) at that time. All screens, including her phone, were banned after the 10 PM alarm sounded. You'll remember from our discussion in the last chapter that I had Stacey buy a good, old-fashioned alarm clock instead of using her phone so she was not tempted to check email or social media first thing upon waking; this is just as important as a tool to avoid checking email "just once more" before falling asleep. I know all too well the disruption of checking email "for the last time," only to find a message from your boss that sends your stress levels through the

SLEEP MACHINES

Just because I think we should ban screens from bedtime doesn't mean I'm not a huge fan of tech that helps us sleep. We are fortunate enough to live in a time when ordinary people are gaining access to amazing sleep technologies and devices, many of them developed for those—like astronauts—who need to get serious sleep while in seriously odd environments. Think about how difficult sleep must be with endless noise, temperature fluctuations, and bad air circulation layered on top of rapidly shifting time zones and a new dawn every ninety minutes! One way these scientists are cracking the sleep code is by using special lighting at night that does not stimulate the brain the way traditional bulbs do. These bulbs are now available for purchase down here on Earth! Look for bulbs that emit red-spectrum light rather than blue. There are apps that change the frequency of light on your devices as well, so that if you must use a screen at night—for instance to read a book—it is at least less disruptive. Another way to make use of this is to switch to a more forgiving light hours before you are ready for bed, to help you wind down.

There are also sleep apps and wearables that can sense our individual sleep cycles. Once these cycles are identified, we can program an alarm to wake us within a range of times, letting the device choose the exact time in the range based upon when we are in the optimal cycle of lighter sleep. Waking in the proper part of your sleep cycle can make rising easier and lead to more energy all day. Need to block out noise? Not only are there are a host of white-noise apps, now there are apps programmed to emit sound at the best frequency for listening to while falling asleep. When sound is too loud, it can be disruptive; too soft, and we are suddenly alert and straining to hear it like a faucet dripping in the background.

From bulbs to apps to wearables to alarms that wake us with gradually brightening natural light, technology doesn't have to be the enemy of sleep—*if* you use it wisely.

roof. That is a surefire sleep killer. And guess what? Your email will still be there in the morning. If it isn't urgent enough for someone to call or show up pounding on your door, it can absolutely wait. We have gotten into the habit of signing over our nonwork hours to our jobs, but I am betting you do not get paid so much that it is worth sacrificing your health.

Stacey found triggering her new routine was critical. Each night when the alarm went off, she was taken completely by surprise and had trouble shutting things down because she "wasn't quite finished." As the weeks went on, it became easier and easier, both to remember the alarm was coming and to shut down when it did. Dimming the lights, taking her magnesium supplement, and turning off the screens helped Stacey get to bed on time, fall asleep more quickly, and experience better-quality sleep. We improved things further by adding logical rules like if she was working on her laptop, she should turn off the TV, and vice versa. To control triggers to eat, Stacey started DVRing her favorite shows so that she saw fewer commercials while watching TV, and she began turning off the lights in her kitchen after 8 PM. Along with alarms on her phone, we used sticky notes around the apartment to remind her not to bring screens into bed, to turn down certain lights, and to stop eating. The new routine, although difficult to adjust to at first, gave Stacey the immediate rewards of more energy, less stress, and increased weight loss.

Many clients stumble by thinking of sleep as only a nighttime consideration. It isn't! Bedtime routines are a perfect place to start, but the changes we made to Stacey's morning routine—getting up earlier, easing into the day with relaxation, using a "real" alarm clock—all supported her ability to get more sleep at night. Just like your diet or hydration, sleep requires planning and awareness throughout your day: what you eat, how much you exercise, how much caffeine you drink . . . all of these things affect sleep.

You can use the following worksheet to plot out your sleep goals and make them a reality.

SLEEP WORKSHEET

If you aren't sure how much sleep you're getting or have trouble answering these questions, I recommend that you track your sleep for three to four nights by simply jotting down what time you go to bed and when you get up, and any notes you have about how you feel or how you slept.

On average, how many hours per night do you sleep?

_____

When you awaken you are . . . (circle one)

RESTED AND READY FOR THE DAY   SLUGGISH AND HITTING SNOOZE   GROGGY AND GROUCHY

Three small shifts I could make to my evening routine to get more sleep or improve my sleep quality would be:

1. _____

2. _____

3. _____

Continued . . .

SLEEP WORKSHEET (CONTINUED)

To trigger each of these small shifts, I will do the following:

1. _____

2. _____

3. _____

Use the shifts you decided upon above and the following chart to outline your new nighttime routine. Record everything: when you will eat, how and when you will begin winding down by dimming or turning off lights and changing into sleepwear, when you'll stop drinking water, etc. Put this somewhere you can see it and practice this routine for several nights in a row to help it stick.

6:00 PM: _____

6:30 PM: _____

7:00 PM: _____

7:30 PM: _____

8:00 PM: _____

8:30 PM: _____

9:00 PM: _____

9:30 PM: _____

10:00 PM: _____

10:30 PM: _____

11:00 PM: _____

11:30 PM: _____

12:00 AM: _____

TYING THE TARGETS TOGETHER

I hold an intense boot camp in my backyard periodically for small groups, introducing the concepts and strategies of Target 100 over the course of ten weeks. I start most sessions by asking members to share what they've been working on that week and how it's affecting their lives, and during a recent check-in, one member, Amy, chimed in to say that, as she pushed for greater awareness in each of the targets, she'd suddenly realized balance was the foundation of the whole program. We begin by focusing on one thing at a time, but eventually it becomes about balancing our efforts among all six targets and understanding the way they work together—and this, not mastering any one area individually, is what makes Target 100 work long term. I couldn't have said it better myself. Balancing focus on all the targets relieves so much of the anxiety associated with the weight-loss process because it makes everything easier and thus more sustainable. The targets are intricately connected—you can look at any single target and see how it affects the others and is affected by them in turn.

To use the subject of this chapter as an example, it is clear that our sleep will never come as easily into line without considering the other targets as well.

Sleep needs . . .

Exercise and movement. Studies show that sleep is radically improved with regular exercise. This isn't rocket science: you've probably noticed that if you tire yourself out doing yardwork, you'll fall asleep more easily that night. Exercise and movement also reduce stress, help alleviate the aches and pains of sitting at a desk all day, increase levels of feel-good hormones like serotonin, and stabilize blood sugar—all things that support your shut-eye.

Sleep needs . . .

A healthy, low-sugar diet. Carb-heavy foods cause blood-sugar spikes and disrupt our natural metabolism and sleep cycles. Overeating can cause reflux, heartburn, or gastrointestinal issues that wake us in the night. Getting enough protein and managing the timing and amount of our alcohol and caffeine consumption can all affect sleep—we can enhance sleep further when we stop eating two hours before bedtime.

Sleep needs . . .

Hydration. Dehydration can make us feel agitated or anxious, and wake us with thirst or muscle cramps. It can cause problems with digestion or lead to poor eating that in turn interferes with rest in the ways discussed above. It can deprive us of the energy we need for sleep-supporting exercise. More directly, remember that water makes up 73 percent of your brain: being dehydrated can disrupt normal brain functions while sleeping. Staying hydrated during the day and then avoiding water for the two hours before bedtime can go a long way toward helping you sleep through the night.

Sleep needs . . .

Stress relief. If we do not address our stress levels, sleep will continue to be a struggle. Stress undermines our good intentions and drives us to sugary foods that wake us in the night. Adrenaline and cortisol pumping through our systems make it impossible to rest, and anxiously churning minds that can't turn off lead inevitably to insomnia. You can't learn to sleep well without learning to relax.

I hope that over the course of looking at these six targets together, you've learned something that has changed your perspective. I have watched so many fall prey to the magical thinking that promises that the latest fad diet will finally be "the thing" that works. I did it (many times) myself. I understand the appeal of narrowing your focus when it comes to weight loss: removing decisions and temptations can feel really good in the beginning. Finally, you don't have to *think* so much! We have become so overwhelmed with options that it feels easier and safer to just take a bunch of those options off the table. With Target 100 I am asking you to do exactly the opposite of narrowing your focus: I want you to broaden your awareness. Expand your idea of what weight loss looks like to include factors you never considered before. What do you have to lose by trying something new? With well over 65 percent of our country overweight or obese, what we are doing now is obviously not working. The simplistic equation of "eat less and move more" is not working, and drastic "quick fix" solutions are not working either, because neither address the whole picture of why the weight crept on to begin with. This physically and emotionally harmful cycle has got to stop. I am asking you to be brave enough to view your body as a fully functioning system, one that doesn't need punishment, but instead requires care. We spend so much time caring for others— it's time to start caring for ourselves.

STRESS · NUTRITION · MOVEMENT · EXERCISE · HYDRATION · SLEEP

HABIT LIBRARY

1. Get new bedding—buy sheets that feel cool against your skin, find a breathable comforter or mattress pad, or try a weighted blanket.
2. Try turning the thermostat down a few degrees more at night.
3. Begin dimming lights two hours before bedtime.
4. Set an alarm to remind you to head to bed thirty minutes early.
5. Remove screens from the bedroom.
6. Stop using your phone as an alarm.
7. Try nighttime yoga or meditation.
8. Keep a glass of water next to your bed so that you don't have to go to the kitchen if you wake up thirsty.
9. Read before bed instead of watching TV.
10. Burn a calming scented candle—like lavender—before bed.
11. Find comfortable sleep clothes.
12. Try a sound machine.
13. Try natural sleep aids like chamomile tea or a magnesium drink before bed.
14. Try using new tech: a wearable device to track and monitor sleep, a wearable alarm to wake you in the best sleep cycle, or an alarm that wakes you gradually with natural light.
15. Take a bath before bed.
16. Create a sleep schedule, and go to bed and wake up at the same time for a full week.
17. Stop eating two hours before bedtime.
18. Add room-darkening shades or drapes.
19. Invest in better pillows/mattress.
20. Clean and organize your bedroom so it is free of chaos.
21. Get outside into natural light at least once every day (going to and from the car doesn't count).
22. Stop drinking caffeine at 2 PM.
23. Try limiting alcohol to before or during dinner.
24. Use your bed only for sleep and sex.
25. Keep a sleep diary to uncover your sleep issues, then make a plan to address one at a time.

TARGETING TOOLS

SUPPORT AND TECHNOLOGY

Chapter 10

YOU NEED A NETWORK

My life was a broken record of fifteen years of failed weight-loss attempts until I discovered the magic of support. It wasn't as if I hadn't tried programs that offered support before: In fact, as a teenager, I was enrolled in one called Diet Center that included weekly weigh-ins and one-on-one sessions with a private counselor. I never took advantage of these benefits or paid any attention to the various "meetings" on offer; I looked at this and every diet system purely as a set of rules to follow. What I missed at the time was that the secret of these types of programs—the whole point of them, really—was the support. I spent many years riffling through diet books, buying fitness videos by the armful, and trying all kinds of weight-loss programs, always on my own. I was an island. I lived inside my head, where my failures seemed epic and a voice whispered that I was broken. I am writing this chapter in the hopes of sparing someone, even one person, the frustration and pain of those years.

I am not going to make you do anything you don't want to do. I won't force you to attend support-group meetings or demand you sign up for a family fitness class, but I will urge you to find your own kind of support— whatever works for you. Support comes in so many forms. It could be an online support group of friends on Facebook, or strangers from a message board, or a group you meet at your gym, or simply one or two of your closest friends. Wherever you find it, community is *huge*. There is an essential human desire to belong, to have people we can relate to and share ourselves with. All of the most successful and lasting wellness brands recognize the importance of feeling like you are part of a group—that someone is with you, watching you, and cares about you. It helps you to show up, which in my experience is half the battle. A diet system is a diet system is a diet system. Don't underestimate how important the support piece is and will be for your long-term success. Who cares if you lose twenty pounds in six weeks if you have to lose the same twenty pounds again six months from now? Support is one of the tools that will make your results the kind that last.

ENVIRONMENT, AGAIN

We've talked a lot about how our environment impacts our habits and behavior, but there is a specific aspect of environment I want to revisit here, and that is the people in it. Some of the spread of the obesity epidemic can be explained by research proving that those we spend time with affect our waistline. As obesity has become more common, it is increasingly likely that every one of us has a friend or family member who is severely overweight. One study, published in the *New England Journal of Medicine*, looked at social networks over a thirty-two-year period, concluding that your friends and family have a huge impact on your biological and behavioral tendency toward obesity. According to the study, if a friend becomes obese, your chances of doing the same increase by 57 percent. In pairs of adult siblings, if one sibling becomes obese, the chance that the other will as well increases by 40 percent. If your spouse becomes obese, the likelihood that you will follow increases by 37 percent. This shouldn't be surprising. These close interpersonal relationships affect us deeply.

Being obese isn't a moral failing, and no one is suggesting that you make weight a prerequisite for friendship. You can be overweight and a shining example of healthy habits, or a svelte, unhealthy couch potato. My point is simply this: Those we spend the most time with help us create and sustain our habits, be they healthy or unhealthy. For example, my sister and I have been each other's greatest allies and greatest handicaps. Some of our worst habits were ones we created together as children. We related to one another through food. Our fondest childhood memories were of secret trips to the local drug store, to buy candy we'd sneak home to eat in bed together late at night. In our college years, we couldn't have a good time unless we were overeating and/or overdrinking. As we grew older and wiser, we worked to unravel those patterns, and now we try valiantly to be our best, healthiest selves together, supporting one another as we pursue our goals. My sister uses me as an accountability buddy to report completing her exercise each day. I rely on her amazing listening skills when I need to talk through behavior patterns I can't seem to shake (and her advice has more than once been the key to changing them). No one knows me quite the way she does. My husband and I, too, can push each other to greatness or drive each other right off the road. We have run marathons together, created a healthy home for our sons, and hope to be strong and fit well into our old age. We also love to eat and drink together, sharing leisurely meals when we travel, trying new things and experimenting in the kitchen. We choose mostly whole, fresh foods and avoid those that are processed or sugary—but if my husband decides to indulge with food or drink, coming home with ice cream or ordering another cocktail while we're out, I have a hard time resisting (even if I've already had an indulgence of my own). I am sure this dynamic will be familiar to every couple. Eating vegetables with hummus while the person next to you on the couch is inhaling kettle chips is a challenge fit for Hercules.

Not all the research about weight and our social networks is discouraging. Involving the most important people in your life in this process can result in better results for all of you. Studies confirm that joining a weight-loss group or starting a weight-loss program *with a friend* drastically increases your odds of success. As we begin to look at weight loss as a game, the people in your immediate circle become your team. Knowing that you will do better if you include others in the process, whom will you invite along? Who are your greatest allies? Which relationships encourage your *un*healthiest habits? Could you open a conversation with those people about making a change? It doesn't have to be hard! "I am trying to lose weight, and whenever we meet at Favorite Restaurant, I end up eating a pile of pita chips. Can we go somewhere else?" Your friends and family should be supportive of your goals. What I see with clients and know from my own experience is that most are suffering in silence alone and don't have any idea how to open a conversation about weight loss. Talking about weight is taboo—we are in a strange place as a culture, where we are supposed to be comfortable with our bodies just the way they are, while thinness is still held up as the ideal. It is OK to want to change or live a healthier life, but many worry that they will offend someone by talking about their wellness goals—in a way they would never worry about discussing their goals in another area. Sometimes people don't want to share because they have failed in the past and don't want to mention that they're trying to lose weight until they feel sure they are actually going to succeed. I urge you to help reshape the conversation about weight and weight management by talking about your goals and your outcomes with others. When we open the conversation about what we want for our lives, without judgment, fear, or shame, walls come down.

THE MAGIC OF ASKING FOR HELP

A common thread among the most successful people I know is their willingness to openly seek out support. They recognize what they are great at and where they could benefit from the help of others, and they actively look for teachers, coaches, or partners who can take them further. They have no fear or shame or hang-ups about getting the help they need: They want to be the best they can be, and they know that this help is what will get them there. When I was invited to Jessica Simpson's wedding, I was seated at what she lovingly called the "guru" table. I sat next to coaches, fitness trainers, meditation experts, and more—amazing people who'd taught either Jess or her husband, Eric, something that enabled them to thrive in a certain area of their lives. I encourage all of my clients to practice seeking support for whatever they need, from career mentorship to cooking, whether from family or friends or professionals. I'll bet you are surrounded by people with skills that could help you or interests you share that you could work on together. Therapists and experts are great, but help doesn't have to be expensive or traditional; it can be whatever fits your life.

For example: After a major move and a big step up for his career, one of my dearest friends, Zach, found himself gaining weight and unable to get around to joining, much less regularly visiting, a new gym. He decided to try a streaming exercise service instead, and start doing one of their ninety-day programs in his basement in the mornings before work. He mentioned this to his neighbor, who asked if he could join him. Before long, some of the other neighbors found out and started showing up. Zach loved it, and it made him accountable: He couldn't decide to sleep in and skip a workout, because he knew a bunch of guys would be showing up on his doorstep bright and early. Together, they all lost weight and got in shape. Zach's basement has become the place to be: Even when he is away on work trips,

Knowing when you need help, how to find help, and how to ask for it are key, not just in weight loss but in all of life. Get a coach, find a guru, or follow an expert. Lean on the people who love you. The habit of asking for help is one of the most powerful you can develop.

the rest of the guys still gather there to work out together! Turning your basement into the neighborhood gym isn't for everyone, but it's what worked for Zach. The point is, don't feel you have to be anything but yourself. Find support in whatever way is right for you.

At first, with private coaching clients, I often found myself perplexed that they weren't reaching out to me more often. As a part of the service, I offer 24/7 access for questions, advice, or just a meal idea when inspiration is running low. I always give clients my phone number and email—they can text me, send me a Facebook message, you name it, but it was rarely happening. That's when I realized most didn't know how to ask for help or use the support I was offering. Many said they felt "shy" about reaching out or reluctant to "bother" me. *Bother* me? I love my job and helping people is what I live for. Hearing from my clients makes me happy: It means they are engaged and working hard, pursuing their goals!

Once I realized that asking for help was something so many clients struggled with, I began teaching it as a habit. Using the habit loop, we began setting reminders and triggers to reach out for support. We examined the feelings and thought patterns that were standing in their way. I began reaching out to clients myself, especially in the early days of our work together, to prove I really was available and could be a valuable resource. Many people don't like asking for help because they believe it is just easier and more efficient to do things themselves, or that they "should" be able to handle a given situation on their own. My male clients seem particularly prone to this type of thinking, but it affects lots of us. When it comes to weight loss, there's often an additional layer of embarrassment or shame. This is a huge problem, but also an opportunity: By practicing asking for help and not shutting down offers of help when they arrive, we can build these behaviors into habits, just like any others. Remember, guilt and shame activate the brain's reward system—work hard to eradicate them.

NEGATIVE SELF-TALK AND THE PLOMS

I see two habitual thought patterns get in the way of people's success time after time, and both are positively impacted by support. One is negative self-talk, and the other is something my mom calls "the PLOMs," as in "Poor Little Old Me"! Negative self-talk is that voice in your head that always has something discouraging or just plain nasty to say about you and your efforts. Those of us who have struggled with our weight tend to be pretty mean to ourselves, often without even realizing it. We may compare ourselves to others and put down our progress, undermine our efforts with cruel reminders of past failures, or simply hear things that are not being said (for instance, hearing "that dress is super flattering on you" as "you need all the help you can get to look presentable"). We have a sort of running commentary of automatic thoughts playing in the back of our minds, thoughts we are barely aware of. I think of it like a radio turned down low—when you're having a conversation with a friend, you might not even notice the background noise, but if you choose to tune in to it, it is there. I remember finally understanding this concept after a friend gave me a compliment about my weight loss, and inside my head I heard myself say, "Thanks for the compliment, but I still look like crap and have a long way to go." I simply couldn't accept the compliment, or acknowledge the progress I had made. Listening to those defeating messages all day is grueling. It eats away at any confidence or positivity we may feel. That voice tricks us into quitting when we hit the first bump in the road, or talks us out of starting in the first place. It says there is no use in trying because we have failed in the past, and anyway, we have too far to go; it will be impossible.

Getting support helps immensely, especially if it gives you the chance to listen to others as they talk about their own struggles. You may not be able to identify your own negative self-talk at first, but you'll definitely hear it in others. You will hear a woman you admire put herself down and say things about herself that you wouldn't say to your worst enemy. She will talk about how certain she is that she will fail and that nothing will ever change. This woman, whom you have been silently emulating, will shock you. You will tell her not to be so hard on herself, that she is doing great . . . and then you will realize that you rarely, if ever, give yourself that same encouragement. You will begin to notice how you speak to yourself, and consciously work to combat the vicious and unhelpful thoughts that crop up. I still hear these thoughts from time to time, but now I simply say to myself "thanks, that's *totally unhelpful*" and move on. I have learned to manage and quiet those thoughts by talking about them with others, or using the skill of gratitude to divert my thinking to something I have done well. We can't continue to whip ourselves, believing that it will drive us forward faster. It is counterintuitive, but the opposite is true. My clients are terrified when I ask them to be kind to themselves. They are afraid they will be so nice that they treat themselves to ice cream cones every day. Nope. Believe it or not, the kinder and gentler you are with yourself, the better you will do.

The Poor Little Old Mes (PLOMs) are really just another version of negative self-talk. They also tell you that you will never succeed, that you are doomed to failure, but they focus on how *unfair* this is, how *unfair* it is that you are broken, that you work so hard and never achieve what seems so easy for everyone else. This petulant voice bemoans all the things we "can't" have and how sorry we feel for ourselves. It tells us that we deserve to have everything we want, weight loss *and* unlimited chocolate chip cookies, because we are trying so hard and it is so awful. It struggles to balance saying yes to ourselves sometimes with saying no at others. Talking openly about these feelings takes the wind out of them. Others can be encouraging and even provide a little tough love, letting you know when it sounds like you're having a case of the PLOMs.

These habitual thought patterns will derail every effort you are making, if you let them, but you can break yourself of the habit of negative self-talk. Left alone with these thoughts they become all-powerful, but with support they are put into perspective, and eventually fade.

ACCOUNTABILITY AND TAKING THE BLINDERS OFF

I finally "got" the support concept at age thirty (what can I say, I was a late bloomer) when I went to Weight Watchers at the urging of a friend who was having success there. I attended the first meeting and hated it. I decided I would take the system and just do it on my own, as usual. I told my friend my plan and she made me promise to go back, just one more time, the next week. I agreed, and something interesting started to happen. I knew that I was going to have to get on the scale in front of someone when I returned, so I got pretty serious about sticking with the plan to see if it even worked. I was pretty sure it wouldn't, but I was scared enough of failing in front of other people that I gave it my best effort. This was my first run-in with real accountability. Knowing that someone would be watching motivated me to up my game. I made my way back to the meeting the following week to find a different leader at the front of the room. The woman from the week before had been a sub. For some reason, this leader totally inspired and motivated me. She was about my age, had dealt with similar struggles, and I liked her style. Most importantly, she made me laugh. In the game of weight loss, I had just found my first teammate. I was completely engaged in the meeting and was thrilled when I got on the scale and found I had actually lost weight. Needless to say, I didn't quit after all. Over the course of the next few meetings, I began to make friends. I looked forward to seeing them every week, to hearing about their progress and sharing my own. These meetings got me out of my head. They made me realize that my "crazy" thoughts and behaviors around food were actually pretty universal and nothing to be ashamed of. Honestly, I could have been following *any* diet, but adding support and accountability changed everything for me.

At one point or another, everyone trying to lose weight struggles to see the solutions and choices that are right in front of them. I am not sure why this is, but I've seen it enough to know it happens to all of us. I have had so many people walk into one of my meetings or boot camps with what feels to them like an impossible challenge, some problem they've run up against they are certain there is no way to solve. The others in the group inevitably see the situation so clearly and differently, free as they are of all the negative baggage we bring to our own problems. The group throws out endless ideas, suggesting small changes that might help, possible approaches and resources. It is like a miracle to watch what happens for the person who is struggling. Suddenly they have a pile of options to sift through, new ideas to consider, and they can settle on the strategies that seem realistic for them and walk out with a game plan and the hopeful attitude that fosters success.

There is always another way to look at a problem, but a key ingredient in perspective is often distance. Take the blinders off by speaking up—and not just for the sake of hearing other people's ideas, but for the gift of hearing yourself. It is said that we remember and internalize only about 25 percent of what others say, while we take in over 75 percent of what we say ourselves. Listening is important, but speaking up and discussing your challenges can lead to the greatest learning. Talking things out, or even typing them into an online forum, will illuminate your experience.

SURROUNDING JENNIFER WITH SUPPORT

When I started working with Jennifer Hudson we worked mainly one to one. She was living in Tampa at the time, and I would head down to see her every two weeks or so. As we began to get to know each other, she mentioned that her family had noticed the changes she was making and were asking a lot of questions about how they might do the same—especially her sister. I was thrilled at the prospect of having someone close to Jennifer join her on her journey, because I knew that the more support she had, the better she would do. A few weeks later I needed to go to Chicago for other business, and I reached out to Jennifer's sister, offering to meet with her and get her started on the program while I was in town. She was excited, and we arranged that when I landed in Chicago, I'd head straight to her from the airport. When I texted her to let her know I was on the way, she asked if I minded if a few other family members joined us. "No problem," I said. "How many?" "Fourteen," she responded. "Whoa! OK!"

Fourteen of Jennifer's family members in Chicago got started that day, but all clamored that they knew other family members who would be interested, too. ("How big is this family?" I asked.) Hoping to give a few more of Jennifer's people a chance to join us, I set up another meeting for the following week.

Thirty-five family members showed up. I was thrilled—it felt so special to meet this amazing group, all so inspired by and supportive of Jennifer, all eager to do something together to make the family healthier. Soon after we got those in Chicago going, they told me that other family members—mainly located in Indianapolis and Mississippi—wanted in as well. I flew down and got them started, too—about twenty-five in Indy and twenty in Mississippi. Eventually, the group swelled to a total of *seventy-five people* across the country, working together, texting each other encouragement, sharing recipes, sending supportive videos, and competing with one another. It was simply one of the most exciting times in my career. Seeing an entire extended family change the way they communicated, how they ate together, how they cooked together, and how they celebrated events together was like nothing I had experienced. That strong support network helped Jennifer in more ways than I can count. Family events became like giant support meetings. Their yearly family reunion became a runway show of all the progress they had made. We even appeared on the final season of *Oprah* to inspire others to involve their families. We don't all have large, close families, but I encourage all my clients to build themselves a network of support. Your network can be made up of anyone: friends, neighbors, coworkers, people you meet online, or all of the above. Just like Jennifer, the more support you have, the better you will do.

SEEKING SUPPORT IS JUST A HABIT

Now you understand the importance of getting support, and of finding the *kind* of support that works for you. Great! Unfortunately, seeking support won't come naturally. Most of us have spent most of our lives trying to avoid talking about our weight at all, much less asking for help in this area. You can complete the task of identifying the right support system (or systems), but then you must create the habit of actually using the support and seeking it out. It is a habit you will have to build like any other, and it may be an uncomfortable one. Use your habit loop, and set triggers to remind you to visit your forums, attend your meetings, or make your calls. I often urge clients to set aside time every evening, when they might otherwise be watching TV or doing something else that triggers old eating behaviors, to spend twenty minutes looking for support and inspiration online, whether in a formal group or on social media. I love scrolling Instagram for inspiration, following amazing success stories, food inspirations, and fitness gurus. My feed is filled with interesting tips and tricks, recipes for healthy food and food for thought, and it invariably chases away the idea that I am alone in whatever I am facing.

There are endless ways to find support that bolsters and strengthens you, but if you can, I do recommend seeking out others, whether online or in person, who are *specifically* tackling weight loss. This challenging emotional, mental, and physical battle is best fought with outside eyes and ears for allies. A few options to consider:

- Private in-person coaching
- Online coaching, in groups or alone
- Commercial weight-loss programs that offer support
- Social media support and motivation
- Internet weight-loss communities
- Nonprofit community organizations like the YMCA or local community centers
- Wellness programs through your medical clinic
- Friends and family
- Workplace groups
- Workout buddies and fitness groups

My advice? Keep an open mind, and try them all until you discover what truly helps. You might surprise yourself.

TARGET 100 BOOK CLUBS

As I neared the end of writing this book, I had a vision of people working their way through Target 100 together, in groups across the country. I wanted to provide an easy way for those following the program to connect with others in reading and following Target 100, and even connect with me as well. So, I came up with the idea of Target 100 book clubs—borrowing from the tradition of book clubs in general, or gathering for weekly game nights at a neighbor's house, while also taking advantage of all the amazing tools technology offers us today and building on what we know about the importance of support. If this book is really resonating with you, I am going to encourage you to be brave and do something a little crazy: Call or email your closest friends and ask them to join you. (Remember, you can cycle through all six targets more than once, so you can absolutely do this even if you've been through all six already.) Target 100 meets you where you are, so no matter how diverse your group's challenges, there is no reason you can't work together, cheering one another on in building healthier lives and even losing some weight.

I've stocked Target100Program.com with all the tools you'll need to get started leading your very own Target 100 book club—you can invite friends, set a date to begin, and designate how often you will meet. For each meeting, you will receive special book club materials to guide the discussion, as well as videos from me. If you want to do something bigger and less local, like Jennifer Hudson and her family—no problem: your group can be all on one block or spread across the country, two people or 100. Online you'll find recipes and a community of others, and I encourage you and your club to connect with me on social media. (Thanks to the wonders of technology, I can even visit book clubs via Skype!)

You'll find plenty of additional details on the website, but the idea is simple: Gather your tribe and surround yourself with support. Because research shows that the more often you meet, the better you do, I recommend weekly meetings, with each person weighing in on the day of the meeting itself—but you could also meet biweekly or even monthly, whatever works for your group. You don't have to sign up online at all, if that's not your thing: You can simply follow the ten-week plan outlined earlier in the book, reading a chapter before each meeting. If you've got a scale, some friends, and a place to meet, you've got everything you need. Like everything else about your Target 100 program, your book club should fit you. Make it your own . . . and then write and tell me all about it!

HABIT LIBRARY

1. Tell friends about your goals.
2. Invite a friend over to cook and share a healthy meal.
3. Join a weight-loss Facebook group or create your own.
4. Attend a weight-loss support-group meeting.
5. Ask for help in some small way every day. Seeking support is like a muscle—flex it and it will grow stronger.
6. Ask a friend to attend an exercise class with you.
7. Set an alarm on your phone a couple of evenings a week reminding you to spend twenty minutes in your online support group.
8. Call or text a friend when you feel tempted to make a food decision that you suspect you'll regret.
9. In your group, bring up a challenge you are facing and ask for suggestions.
10. Write down three positive thoughts you have had about yourself recently.
11. Take a compliment without responding with something self-deprecating—and don't allow negative thoughts to erase it.
12. Make a list of areas in your life where you could use a coach.
13. Start a "gratitude jar." When something good happens or you're feeling grateful, write it on a slip of paper and toss it in. Reread these when you need a boost.
14. Tell someone who is not being supportive that you need their help.
15. Talk to a close friend or family member about *why* your goals are important to you.
16. Start a "healthy lunch club" at work.
17. Sign up for a workout class where you will begin to see some of the same people weekly and make like-minded friends.
18. Join an online step challenge with friends or family.
19. Get friends together and create a monthly potluck dinner to share healthy recipes.
20. Support others! Go out of your way to listen and give advice to those who are supporting you.
21. Log on to Target100Program.com to create your own weight-loss group.
22. Place a small notebook by your bedside and write down three things you are grateful for every morning upon waking. (It's a great way to get serotonin flowing in the AM!)
23. Make a list of the most supportive people in your life.
24. Start a walking group at the office—meet daily before or after work, at lunch, or on an afternoon break.
25. Check out events in your community, like 5Ks or wellness classes.

Chapter 11

TECHNOLOGY IS YOUR FRIEND

ow, I am what you might call an "early adopter" when it comes to technology. As one of the very first employees at Weight Watchers Online, Weight Watchers' start-up brand, I had a front-row seat as technology began to transform the world of wellness. The internet was just blossoming, and it was all new to me. I was just over thirty years old and remember vividly being one of the "old" members of the dot com team. My job was to translate the principles of the programs to the engineers building the site. I was surrounded by a bunch of young guys who came to work on skateboards, in shorts. I understood almost none of what they were doing at first, but, to be fair, they understood almost nothing about what I was doing either. They had never followed the program themselves and had no idea how a user would want to see it laid out, what would be most helpful, and what would make it fun to use. We spent hours moving buttons and adjusting pages to make the design more intuitive for someone trying to learn the program completely on their own, and I would go on to spend years developing online tools and content.

This experience opened my eyes to the power of technology. Weight Watchers Online brought the program into the homes of people who otherwise would never have been able to try it because they lived too far from a meeting site—not to mention the millions who had been held back from joining because the meetings intimidated them or didn't fit their schedules. My work with Weight Watchers ended, but what endured is a passion for building tech that can change lives. Today I continue to spend a portion of my time consulting and advising some of the most forward-thinking health and wellness companies—like Misfit wearables—as they develop emerging technologies. Technology has been a game changer for wellness and weight loss, and I am hoping that my passion for this subject will rise off these pages and capture your imagination.

OVERCOMING iPHOBIA

In a very real way, technology has brought the world within reach. Unfortunately, new technology often runs up against some resistance—it's been that way since the printing press. We're habit-driven creatures, after all! Technology can seem particularly intimidating to those, like me, who didn't grow up with computers or cell phones, but even people who are comfortable with tech can be reluctant to do something differently, or just feel overwhelmed by the sea of options we have today. I get it, I do! But give me a chance. I had a record player and a rotary phone, and I promise you, if I can learn to love technology, you can, too. I'm not going to suggest that you learn to program your computer or recommend you buy tons of expensive equipment, I am simply going to take you on a tour of the unique ways existing, easy-to-use technologies can make your weight-loss journey—and your life—easier, and help you on the way to any behavior change you want to make.

Today you can weigh in via a wireless scale that tracks your progress on your smartphone; find support on the internet and social media; use a breathalyzer to measure fat burn; monitor your intake of specific nutrients with apps and your movement and exercise with wearables; investigate your sleep with a sleep monitor; use your phone to meditate and to remind you to meditate. It's a brave new world—but it doesn't have to be that complicated.

In fact, I'll bet you are more tech savvy than you think. Let's do a little questionnaire to help you realize it. If you can answer yes to any three of these questions, you are more than ready to use technology to aid you in your weight-loss efforts:

1. Do you own a computer?
2. Can you access and browse the internet?
3. Have you ever set up a new phone, watch, or even speakers to sync with your computer?
4. Do you own a smartphone?

5. Do you know how to set the alarm on your smartphone?
6. Do you know how to take pictures on your smartphone?
7. Have you ever downloaded and set up an app on your smartphone?

How did you do? That's about the extent of the skills I am asking you to be open to mastering. Little things, like using your phone to take pictures of your meals prior to eating them, can be powerful. Why? By creating this simple habit, you are cataloguing the meals that you love in pictures—any number of one-touch apps will let you collect those photos into an amazing book of your own meals to use for inspiration. What's more, taking a quick photo of your meal makes you more likely to lay it out nicely on a plate, and causes you to pause briefly before eating it. That short pause and focus on the food creates awareness, and can slow you down just enough to help you eat more mindfully and moderately—natural fullness cues set in after a number of minutes, but if you are shoveling your food in quickly, you'll finish before they arrive (or fail to notice them at all). Taking our picture example one step further, you can post your meal on social media or your weight-loss group for support and encouragement of your healthy choices.

Now let's look at how one simple change—like ordering your groceries online—can transform your weight-loss process. In the majority of households today, all adults in the home work. Not only do most of us work, we're working longer hours, alongside juggling record numbers of activities and commitments for our families. The average trip to the grocery store, from start to finish, takes over an hour—often longer. What if, after the initial setup, you could reduce the process to a few clicks of a button, and reclaim that time for your week? In addition to saving time, what is possibly the most tempting place in the world to navigate? You guessed it. We have talked about food cues, decision fatigue, and the secondary hunger system—the grocery store is a land mine! What if you could leave roaming the aisles to someone else? I guarantee it will reduce the amount of junk that makes it into your house. Today's online grocery shopping platforms are wonders of tech genius. They allow you to keep a "standard" list so you don't have to reinvent the wheel every time you shop, and track past purchases so you can reorder with ease. Some work with online recipe sites and allow you to add the ingredients you need right from the recipe page. Some have lovely prepackaged meals available for nights you don't feel like cooking. Nutrition information is available at your fingertips, and the whole order can be delivered to your door. If that's not life-changing technology, I don't know what is.

YOUR SUPERPHONE

The biggest game changer of all is probably sitting next to you right now: your smartphone. Ten years ago, only 6 percent of American adults had smartphones, but as of this writing we're at about 80 percent, and it's a safe bet that we'll approach 100 percent in the next few years. Today our phones are high-powered microcomputers. They are also cameras, social media gateways, internet browsers, music players, and more. The best feature of your smartphone from a habit-building perspective is that you never leave home without it. In fact, it is almost the *only* thing we never leave home without these days. Now, our phones can be our wallet, and in the not-so-distant future, our phones may be our keys as well. Smartphones are—by far—my favorite weight-loss tech tool.

In my time with Weight Watchers, the single greatest breakthrough for members came when we launched our smartphone app. Suddenly, members had a tool with them everywhere they went to track what they ate and to look up nutritional information. With the launch of the app, we saw adherence to the program increase and success rise right alongside it. This makes sense: Just seeing the phone—and the app on it—reminded (i.e., triggered) members to record their food or make smarter choices (i.e., practice their new routine). That added level of consistency gave them better results (and the reward of greater weight loss). Consistency—as I've said, well, *consistently*—is what creates success. Not perfection, but making small changes and sticking with them over the long term.

When clients leave my office with clear goals for the week and the best of intentions, and return having failed to achieve something, it is rarely because it was too difficult or they weren't motivated enough—it's usually because they simply forgot. They forgot to set up the trigger, to leave the sticky note, to try entering their house through a new door. Sometimes we forget things; we are not computers! Luckily, our phones are. Now I have clients set phone reminders before they even leave my office. The fact that your phone is always with you makes it the ultimate triggering tool. For example, when my client Linda was struggling to get into the habit of planning her next day the evening before, we set an alarm on her phone for each night at 8 PM that said: "text Liz." For the next two weeks, she had to text me every evening and briefly outline the next day—highlighting things like what she would be eating and when she would exercise, whether she had social plans or other challenges, and if so, how she would navigate them. This helped Linda to develop the habit of thinking ahead, recognizing when she had overscheduled herself or was likely to run into food troubles the next day.

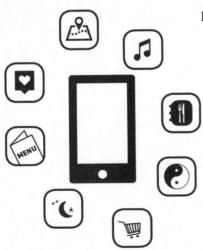

Identifying challenges meant she could plan for them, which resulted in greater consistency in her food and exercise choices—and greater weight loss as a result.

I myself use the alarms and calendar on my phone religiously, and review my schedule for the next day every evening. I schedule and set reminders for my workouts, the walk breaks I take throughout the day, mealtimes, you name it. This ensures that things that are important to me, like stress relief and movement, have a place in my day and don't get pushed to the side. Using my phone to manage and trigger my time has made me more efficient and organized—and remember, chaos, clutter, and even being late can stress us out and lead to poor choices.

I'm not saying your phone is the magic solution to every problem, but I do think it can be an amazing ally.

Let's look at the targets one at a time and consider how your phone might help you take aim at each of them:

Food: My clients all use their phones to Google carb counts, and you can also use a variety of apps that give you nutritional information when you scan a bar code or even take a picture. You can record your carb totals in the notes app or in any number of nutrition apps. Search low-carb recipes online and join related Facebook, Instagram, and Pinterest groups. Take pictures of the foods you eat to keep track and create awareness. Post those pictures to social media for support. Call or text a friend when temptation strikes. Look up restaurants and menus prior to dining out and use apps like Yelp to discover healthy dining options close to wherever you are at the moment.

Water: Staying hydrated is a lot easier when you use your phone to remind yourself to drink up—set alarms every hour or so to refill your water bottle. Get yourself one of the amazing new "connected" water bottles that not only track your intake on an app but also glow when you have left them to sit idle for too long. Use your phone to join in on water challenges, download a free hydration app that sends push notifications to remind you to drink, or just keep track of those 100 ounces somewhere other than your head.

Exercise: Take advantage of streaming exercise options like YouTube, Beachbody, or Daily Burn. There are personal training apps and amazing new services that allow a trainer to see you through a Skype-like platform and lead you in a workout. Use apps like ClassPass to find discounted and open workout classes near you and book your spot right from your phone. There are apps like C25K (Couch to 5k) that get you started on running slowly, and apps that let you track your runs along with time and speed. Download and create amazing workout playlists, too!

Movement: Your phone can serve as a GPS on your walks, letting you plan different routes and track how long (and how far) you go. Wearable fitness trackers sync with your phone and give you oodles of real-time data about your activity level and daily step count. Use your phone to time yourself doing housework or gardening and track your minutes. Set alarms to remind yourself to get up and move every hour during the day.

Stress relief: There are endless apps that offer a wide variety of meditation styles and experiences. Download a breathing-exercise app and use it for a few minutes in the afternoon or whenever you feel most stressed at work. Find a yoga routine on YouTube or set an alarm for a power nap. Use your phone's calendar or other productivity and organization apps to keep you feeling stress free. Book a fifteen-minute rant with your therapist on Skype, or try a guided cognitive behavioral therapy app. Book a massage.

Sleep: Set an alarm to remind you to turn lights down and screens off about thirty minutes before bed. Track sleep minutes and quality through your wearable or even use a sleep-cycle app to analyze its data and wake you gradually in the right part of your sleep cycle. Use your phone as a sound machine to block out noise for better sleep. Try guided meditation to help you relax and fall asleep more quickly. Block the use of certain apps at certain hours to keep you offline if you use your phone for sleep, and use the "Do Not Disturb" function to turn off notifications after a specific time. Switch your screen to a "Nighttime" setting in the evening to avoid stimulating light.

CONNECT FOUR

As it applies to weight loss, I find that technology can be separated into four distinct categories: support and education; devices; services; and tools and apps. To get the most you can out of your tech, experiment with and seek out resources from all four areas.

Support and Education

At the end of the day, I believe the most important benefit of the explosion of technology over the past few decades has been connecting us with others. By doing this, it has also connected us with information: Thanks to the internet, we have an impossibly vast universe of knowledge available to us from virtually anywhere. It is both easier to access experts and easier to become an expert yourself! You can educate yourself by reading and researching on your own, and learn from professionals providing online courses, podcasts, and more. There are forums and podcasts on just about every topic, from meditation to the latest in nutrition science. There is less reason than ever to blindly follow a one-size-fits-all program handed down by a weight-loss expert—you can literally build your own (which is what I am begging you to do with the help of this book!) thanks to the incredible informational resources and support available online. I really leaned on the internet when I had to experiment with a ketogenic diet as a member of the research team for a breath-analysis device. A ketogenic diet is one where you take in only the tiniest amount of carbohydrates while your intake of fat is extremely high—somewhere between 65 and 85 percent of your daily calories. I'd never tried the diet before and I knew I needed to get educated and seek support in order to really master it in a healthy way and make my research as useful as possible. I spent some time watching webinars by doctors and experts at the University of Southern California about the diet itself, read a couple of e-books, and then got involved with the Reddit boards on the subject for support. It was empowering as I embarked on this totally new (and a little intimidating!) experiment to know I could chat with people who had followed the diet themselves; I could watch professionals explain it; follow "Keto" bloggers, and even reach out to them via Facebook or Twitter. I was able to take the journey at my own pace with support available whenever I needed it. I loved the folks on the Reddit boards—it was like a virtual version of my old Weight Watchers meetings.

I know we already had a whole chapter on the subject, but support is one of the most effective weight-loss tools out there. In the simplest terms, we are stronger and more focused in groups of like-minded people. Use technology to bring friends and family along on your journey, even if they are across the world, or use technology to find your "tribe" elsewhere. There isn't a single diet, weight-loss goal, or life situation in general that you can't find support for on the internet, I promise you. Reddit's message boards alone cover just about every subject. The thing I loved about online forums is that someone was always available, 24/7, to listen or offer suggestions. Most importantly, they understood me—because they had been where I was and knew what I was going through.

Devices

From body composition scales and even wirelessly syncing food scales (that enter your food automatically in your tracking app once it is weighed) to sleep monitors, fitness trackers, and stress monitors, devices are giving us data about ourselves that we simply never had before.

These devices can help you define and refine your weight-loss program by showing you just how many steps or how much exercise you need to put

you in the weight-loss "zone."
Let's say you walk 10,000 steps a
day and exercise every weekday.
If you knew that just three days of
exercise on top of 12,000 steps a day
was enough to result in weight loss,
would you still work out five times
a week? Maybe, but maybe not! We
all have varying priorities. Data—not
just from devices, but from tracking apps
in general—can tell you, based on results,
whether you should focus on adding more
yoga or strength training, whether you need
to consume less or more food (really!) to
sustain weight loss. It can help you hone in on your
perfect macronutrient profile—the percentage of fats, carbs, and protein that
not only lets you lose weight but makes you feel your best, too.

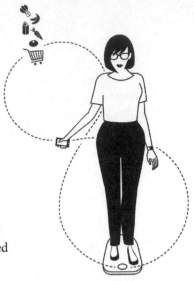

Some advice about devices, however: Give less weight to the numbers
themselves than to the trends they reveal. Numbers don't lie, but one
number alone tells us almost nothing. The important thing isn't *where* you
start, it's that you *do* start, and keep going.

You might remember that when we discussed devices in the movement
chapter I told you that half of all wearable devices sold end up unused.
You buy one full of hope that it will magically make you more active, but
once you are home that hope turns to fear or doubt. What if you are only
getting, like, 200 steps? What if you are the *least active person in the history
of step counters*? How do you even get this thing to talk to your phone?

I have clients break their device purchase into small, distinct tasks so
they don't get overwhelmed (and actually use it):

1. Set aside time to research which device is right for you. Ask friends via
   social media or in person for advice—what do they like and dislike about
   devices they have tried?
2. Schedule a time to order the device online or to visit a store to buy it.
3. Set aside a block of time in your calendar to set up the device and get
   familiar with it and the corresponding app on your phone or computer.
   Most devices come with 24/7 support via chat or phone—take advantage
   of it if you get frustrated! Don't miss out on amazing features because you
   aren't sure how to use them.

4. Set up your profile and reach out to any friends you have in the community of users. The social aspect of any device will make you more likely to use it more often, and "doing" is how transformational learning occurs. You can't learn anything from a device if it's in a drawer.
5. Commit to using your device and looking carefully at your data each week. (If you forget to put it on in the morning at first, or to charge it, set yourself reminders!) Look at the graphs and charts to find patterns in your life, and then use that data to make habit changes. Is your step count particularly low on a certain day every week? Why? How could you change that?

They may not be magic, but the exciting part about the world of devices and wearables is that this is just the beginning. In a few years we will look back and laugh at the giant wristband fitness trackers we wore, because the same technology will be embedded instead in tiny sensors on clothing, in buttons and shoes. We are moving from wearables to forgettables, and as the technology continues to develop, the data we will be able to collect will blow your mind—and help you stay healthier.

Apps and Tools

There really *is* an app for that, whatever *that* is. There are over 50,000 wellness-related apps on the market right now. By the time you read this, that number will certainly be higher. There is an app for anything you might want to track or monitor when it comes to weight loss, health, or habits in general. Best of all, the app world is getting more and more interconnected. The larger players in the field have begun to understand that you, the consumer, might not want to track several different indicators in several different apps, and they have begun working together so that all of your information can be viewed in one place. Platforms like Fitbit, MyFitnessPal, and Lose It! allow you to connect your accounts from multiple apps so that you can see the data you have tracked across them—food eaten, exercise and steps taken, sleep hours, and so on—all in one place. Putting all of this information together can make the light bulb come on. Suddenly you notice that each time you get less than six hours of sleep, you overeat the next day. Or that on days you have a fiber-filled dinner, you are less likely to snack later in the evening. This is the kind of transformational learning we aim for. Seeing for yourself that staying up late leads to you, personally, overeating will do more to convince you that sleep matters for weight loss than anything you read in an article or a book (even this one)!

Apps make amazing behavior-modification tools. Not only are they on your (ever-present) phone, most have push notification systems that can act as the trigger for your new routine, and they often apply gamification principles to keep you motivated and engaged. Additionally, if the larger, more integrated platforms feel overwhelming, there is a singularly focused app for just about any habit you're looking to create, allowing you to concentrate on one new routine at a time. There are apps like Sleep Cycle that use sound to track your sleep cycles—no wearable device needed, this app uses your phone's microphone to analyze your breathing patterns. Apps like Calm help you establish a meditation routine, while apps like Happier can be a gratitude journal and mindfulness aid. Just search the app store for any behavior you are trying to change or cultivate (or just search "habit" for great habit-tracking and motivational apps)—I guarantee you will find something helpful!

Services

No matter what your goals, there are services available via your computer or even your phone to help you achieve them. Some of my favorites to recommend are the new meal-kit delivery services that deliver premeasured ingredients, complete with fresh meat and produce. Many of these now offer total customization, with vegetarian, gluten-free, low-carb, and quick-prep options to choose from. All you have to do is take the ingredients out of the box, do some light prep, and follow the simple, illustrated recipe card—in some cases you just assemble and pop in the oven. The other night I had miso-glazed salmon and veggies steamed in a foil packet with a light sesame-oil sauce, from box to table in half an hour and all made on a single sheet pan. (We have come a long way from the frozen horror show that was "meal delivery" back in the day.) And you no longer have to commit to a particular service for every meal—you can specify the number of days and servings and to skip weeks whenever you like, or even use one service one week and another the next. So many of my clients have gotten back to having healthier meals thanks to these services. It allows them to outsource the time-consuming work of shopping and measuring while preserving the joy of cooking for their families—and it is a great way to get started if you aren't much of a cook or have relied heavily on processed foods.

I am also a huge fan of streaming exercise services. For many, the extra fifteen to twenty minutes driving to and from a gym, on top of their workout time, is more than they have to give. Lots of exercise programs—everything from barre classes and ballet-inspired workouts to high-intensity interval training—have streaming services that bring the studio to you, and streaming platforms like Netflix, Hulu, and Amazon have exercise offerings as well. What's more, many people don't realize that they may have *free* exercise-on-demand services already, right on their television or cable box. These services offer an amazing variety of options for whatever amount of time you have available. Have just ten extra minutes in the morning? Stream a ten-minute yoga class right into your living room (and it's free)! You can use YouTube the same way.

Many coaches and personal trainers now offer their services virtually—I love that technology allows me to reach clients across the world for consultations via Skype or Google Hangouts. You can find online help for whatever you struggle with, whether it is diet or stress relief. Today there are therapists and sleep experts, financial planners, meditation gurus, and even personal assistants offering their services remotely.

THRIVING IN A TECH-FUELED WEIGHT-LOSS WORLD

The key to incorporating tech into your plan is to be just as task-oriented as you would be in any other area. For whatever behavior you are working on, take the time to seek out possibilities in each of the four segments we have discussed here. Do you need more information and education? Where is the community of support? Is there a device to help you gather data? A tool or app that could assist you? Can you find a service associated with it? The answer to all of these is likely to be yes, so it's important to remember that each of these uses may be new for you, and will need to be approached like any other habit. Don't try to do everything at once! To start, think of just three small things you would like to do to fold technology into your plan.

THREE SMALL THINGS I WILL DO THIS WEEK TO INCORPORATE TECH INTO MY PROGRAM

1. _____

2. _____

3. _____

Three small tasks—like downloading an app, setting a timer, or making a shared grocery list on your phone.

Technology can be a huge asset, once you know how to take advantage of it. Check the Habit Library for ideas, take whatever inspires you, and make it your own. Have fun with it! I was a complete tech newbie at thirty, and now it is a huge part of my life—you never know what will spark something in you.

I'll leave you with a snapshot of my very own tech-fueled day.

5:00 AM: My "gentle wake" app soothes me into my day. I strap my Fitbit around my wrist so I get every last step I can! Then I check in on how much and how well I slept the night before with the Beddit sleep-monitor app.

5:45 AM: The first client arrives in my gym. I use my phone as a timer for circuits and stream inspirational music to fuel the workout.

7:00 AM: I check my weather app to decide what my own workout will be. If it's rainy or cold, I stream something from Beachbody. I use my meditation app for a quick ten-minute session before I head into the rest of my day.

8:00 AM: I step on my wireless body-composition scale to check in on my weight and body-fat percentage, and take a look at the graph of my trends. Then I walk my kids to school to get some quality time with them (and get more steps)!

9:00 AM: I make a quick, easy breakfast and track it in the Lose It! app on my phone.

10:00 AM: Work time in my office, using my phone alarm to remind me to drink water and get up and move a bit every hour. Lunch is usually leftovers from the night before, eaten around 12:30.

2:30 PM: Walk to pick up my kids from school for a little more quality time with them (and more steps for me)! Get the kids a snack and set them up for the afternoon. Get myself a snack and track it!

3:00 PM: Continue working from home.

5:30 PM: Begin prepping one of the Blue Apron meals that are delivered to my doorstep once a week.

6:30ish PM: Sit down with the kids for a healthy dinner together.

7:00 PM: Homework time. I help the kids, but I also spend a little time on *my* homework: I take a few minutes to think through the next day's schedule and what my meals will look like. If it's a meal-planning day, I browse for healthy recipes and inspiration for the week. I set any reminder alarms I may need. I spend a few minutes on social media looking through posts from my "tribe," and I spend a few minutes on Reddit boards or other communities keeping up with what is going on in my field.

8:00 PM: Settle in to binge-watch a couple of episodes of my current favorite show. I take a break between episodes to stretch and get the kids to bed.

9:30 PM: An alarm goes off to remind me to turn down lights, turn off screens, and get ready for bed. I head upstairs for a little "me time" with a book.

10:00 PM: Time for some shut-eye. I set my alarm on my phone . . . and place it across the room so I can't check it again! If I have trouble falling asleep, I turn on a guided meditation or sound-machine app to help me relax, then put my phone back in its place, using the sleep function so it will turn off automatically. Zzzzzzz . . .

HABIT LIBRARY

1. Set alarm to remind you to begin your bedtime routine.
2. Download a new stress-relief app.
3. Block off fifteen minutes on your phone calendar for meditation and set up a notification to remind you of your appointment with yourself.
4. Set up grocery delivery.
5. Download three new songs to your workout playlist.
6. Download a nutrition app.
7. Spend ten minutes scrolling through weight-loss and recipe Pinterest boards for inspiration and motivation.
8. Set an alarm to remind you to refill your water bottle midway through the day.
9. Join the Target 100 Facebook group for support.
10. Research wearable wellness devices.
11. Purchase or set up your wearable device.
12. Join a challenge group with your wearable device for some accountability and motivation.
13. Set up a sleep monitor.
14. Explore the fitness videos available on YouTube.
15. Begin taking pictures of your meals.
16. Use your phone as a GPS and distance tracker for your run or walk.
17. Try a healthy meal-delivery service like Blue Apron or HelloFresh.
18. Purchase a wireless scale that syncs with your phone.
19. Find a blogger or two in a self-improvement area that interests you and follow them.
20. Try a streaming exercise service like Daily Burn. (Most have thirty-day free trials.)
21. Download a hydration app.
22. Search social media for, and follow, inspirational people who share your interests. Fill your feed with motivation!
23. Explore the Reddit boards under "weight loss."
24. Set an alarm that reminds you to get out for a ten-minute walk twice a day to relieve stress and keep your metabolism humming.
25. Watch a free webinar on nutrition, or another wellness-related topic that you'd like to learn more about.

RECIPES

H ere are ten of my favorite easy, low- or low-ish-carb recipes for those of you who could use some mealtime inspiration.

Cooking to cover multiple meals at once is a great way to make healthy eating easier on hectic schedules. Some people find it useful to do much of their prep and cooking for the week on the weekend. When I cook, I like to make that cooking time really count by making "extra." Sometimes I use leftovers for lunches or another meal, but often I use them to make something that is entirely new, but takes even less effort.

Each of these recipes is designed to leave you with leftovers, and for each recipe here you'll find two additional complete recipes, designed to make use of these leftovers, online at Target100Program.com. I've included some less formal suggestions for leftovers here as well.

GRILLED PORK TENDERLOIN WITH ONIONS AND PEPPERS

SERVES 4 PLUS LEFTOVERS

Turning the pork 3 times on the grill ensures that it is evenly charred and cooked through. After each 5-minute interval, simply roll the tenderloins so a raw side faces the flame.

Use leftovers to make one of these additional recipes, available online:

- Tex Mex Salad
- Pork Fajitas

Other ideas for leftovers:

- Simmer leftover peppers in marinara sauce with some pitted olives. Add sturdy white fish fillets and poach in the sauce until cooked through. Top with chopped basil.

- For 4 servings, chop a leftover pork tenderloin and half of the peppers and onions. Toss with 1 cup of your favorite grain (like bulgur) or couscous and dress with lemon juice, olive oil, and fresh herbs. Add crumbled feta or goat cheese, if you like.

....

Juice of 1 lime, plus wedges for serving
1 tablespoon chili powder
2 teaspoons ground cumin
¼ teaspoon granulated garlic
4 tablespoons extra virgin olive oil, divided
Kosher salt
2 boneless pork tenderloins (about 1¼ pounds each)
4 medium bell peppers (any colors), stemmed, seeded, and quartered
2 large onions, peeled and sliced into ½-inch rings

1. Preheat an outdoor grill or large 2-burner grill pan or griddle to medium heat.
2. In a small bowl, stir together the lime juice, chili powder, cumin, granulated garlic, and 3 tablespoons of the olive oil until smooth. Season the pork tenderloins lightly with salt and toss with half of this marinade. Brush the peppers and onions with the remaining tablespoon of olive oil, season with salt, and rub with the remaining marinade.
3. Grill pork tenderloins for 5 minutes. Roll the tenderloins over to the next side and cook 5 minutes more. Roll one more time and cook until just pink in the center (you can cut into one to check) or until an instant-read thermometer inserted in the center registers 145 degrees, about 8 to 12 minutes more, depending on size. Remove the pork to a cutting board and let rest 10 minutes while you grill the vegetables.
4. Add the vegetables to the grill and cook, turning once or twice, until tender and charred in places, about 6 to 8 minutes. Remove the vegetables as each is done.
5. Reserve half of the vegetables and pork for later. Slice the remaining pork and coarsely slice or chop the vegetables. Serve with lime wedges.

About 9 grams of carbs per serving (¼ of a pork tenderloin plus ⅛ of the peppers and onions)

HERB ROASTED CHICKEN WITH GREENS

SERVES 4 PLUS LEFTOVERS

Remove the top rack of the oven and roast the chickens on the bottom rack. The heat from the bottom of the oven will caramelize the pan juices and add great flavor to the greens! Three bunches of greens may seem like a lot, but they cook down more than you think. Buy whatever is on sale and looks fresh, and don't be afraid to mix varieties—spinach, kale, chard, collards, etc.

Use leftovers to make one of these additional recipes, available online:

- Creamy Chicken Salad with Apples and Pecans
- Slow-Cooker Chicken Noodle Soup

Other ideas for leftovers:

- Simmer diced chicken and greens in marinara or other tomato sauce, adding ¼ cup cooked white beans, for a quick stew. Sprinkle with grated Parmesan before serving.
- Toss diced chicken and greens with marinated artichoke hearts, diced fresh mozzarella, and halved cherry tomatoes for a quick antipasto-style salad.

....

4 tablespoons unsalted butter, at room temperature
2 cups loosely packed fresh basil leaves
1 cup loosely packed fresh Italian parsley leaves
1 lemon, zested and halved
Kosher salt
Freshly ground black pepper
2 (4- to 4½-pound) whole chickens
1 head garlic, smashed into cloves
Water
3 large bunches greens of your choice (kale, spinach, or Swiss chard), washed and coarsely chopped
Splash of cider vinegar or other vinegar

1. Preheat oven to 425 degrees. Place a rack in a roasting pan large enough to hold the chickens side by side.
2. With a fork, mash the butter, basil, parsley, lemon zest, ½ teaspoon salt, and some pepper in a small bowl to make a paste (or puree in a food processor). Rub the paste all over the chickens and under the skin of the breasts, and season each lightly with salt and pepper. Squeeze a lemon half over each chicken and stick a squeezed-out half into each chicken

cavity. Peel and slice 2 of the garlic cloves and reserve. Divide the rest of the unpeeled cloves between the cavities of the two chickens.

3. Arrange the chickens on the rack so that they are next to each other, but not touching. Pour about 1 cup water in the bottom of the pan. Roast the chickens, basting with the pan juices 3 times and adding water ½ cup at a time as needed to keep the bottom of the pan from burning, until the skin is crisp and golden and the temperature registers 165 degrees on an instant-read thermometer, about 1 hour and 15 minutes, depending on the size of the chickens. (If you don't have a thermometer, the chicken is done when the leg wiggles easily and the juices of the thigh run clear.) Remove the chickens from the roasting pan and let rest on a cutting board.

4. On a burner over medium heat, add the sliced garlic to the juices remaining in the roasting pan and cook until sizzling, about 1 minute. Add all of the greens and season with 1 teaspoon salt and some pepper. Stir to coat the greens in the pan juices. Cook, stirring occasionally, until the greens are wilted and tender, about 6 to 8 minutes. Add a splash of vinegar.

5. Carve 1 chicken into pieces and serve with the greens. Reserve the other chicken and 1 cup of greens for other recipes.

About 9 grams of carbs per serving (¼ of a chicken plus ¾ cup greens)

ITALIAN MEATBALL CASSEROLE

SERVES 4 PLUS LEFTOVER MEAT MIXTURE

Most grocery stores sell meatloaf mix that is a mixture of beef, pork, and veal, but you can also use ground beef alone. The carb count for jarred marinara or other tomato-based sauces can vary widely (depending on how much sugar is added!), so look at the label if you aren't making your own. A good brand with just a few fresh ingredients can have as few as 4 grams of carbs per serving.

Serve this casserole with a green salad or steamed broccoli on the side.

Use leftovers to make one of these additional recipes, available online:

- Open-Face Mushroom Burgers
- Mini Meatloaves with Quick Pan Gravy and Mashed Cauliflower

Other ideas for leftover meatball mixture:

- Brown half of the raw mixture in a skillet with olive oil and add a jar of sauce for a chunky meat sauce for zucchini or spaghetti squash noodles.

- Form the mixture into ovals and press onto skewers. Brush with oil, and grill. Serve over a green salad with tomatoes, mozzarella, and balsamic vinaigrette.

....

1 medium onion, cut into chunks
1 medium carrot, peeled and cut into chunks
3 cloves garlic, crushed and peeled
2½ pounds meatloaf mix (or ground beef)
½ cup plus 2 tablespoons grated Parmesan
½ cup dry bread crumbs
2 large eggs, beaten
2 teaspoons dried Italian seasoning
Kosher salt
Freshly ground black pepper
1 tablespoon extra virgin olive oil
¼ cup water
2 cups prepared marinara
1¼ cups grated mozzarella

1. Preheat oven to 425 degrees.
2. In a food processor, pulse the onion, carrot, and garlic until finely chopped.
3. In a large bowl, combine the meat, onion-carrot-garlic purée, ½ cup grated Parmesan, the eggs, bread crumbs, Italian seasoning, 2 teaspoons salt, and a generous grinding of black pepper. Mix well with your hands. Wrap and refrigerate half of the mixture for another recipe.
4. Brush the bottom of a 9×13-inch glass or ceramic baking dish with the olive oil. Form the meat mixture into 16 meatballs and arrange in the dish.
5. Stir ¼ cup water into the marinara sauce. Pour the marinara over the meatballs and into the baking dish. Sprinkle with the mozzarella and the remaining 2 tablespoons of grated Parmesan. Cover with foil and bake until the meatballs are cooked through, about 15 minutes. Uncover and bake until the cheese is browned and bubbly, about 5 to 7 minutes more.

About 15 grams of carbs per serving (4 meatballs plus sauce)

PESTO SHRIMP WITH ZUCCHINI "NOODLES"

SERVES 4 PLUS LEFTOVERS

Fresh pesto is easy and quick to make, but you can also use a good-quality prepared pesto here—you'll need about ½ to ¾ cup. I haven't put Parmesan in this pesto, because we're using it on seafood, but you can stir in ¼ cup grated Parmesan if you like.

The "spiralizer" is a relatively new gadget used to make noodles from all sorts of vegetables. You can also now purchase vegetables "pre-spiralized" in the produce section of larger supermarkets.

Use leftovers to make one of these additional recipes, available online:
- Shrimp Salad Stuffed Tomatoes
- Greek Salad with Pesto Shrimp

Other ideas for leftovers:
- If you have a few tablespoons of leftover pesto, it is delicious stirred into vegetable soups at the end of their cooking time. You can also toss roasted vegetables in a few tablespoons of pesto once they're out of the oven, or brush pesto on fish fillets or chicken breasts before grilling, baking, or broiling.
- Leftover shrimp is great sautéed with spinach or other quick-cooking greens. Top with a little Sriracha or other hot sauce.

....

¼ cup pine nuts or skinned almonds
2 cups loosely packed fresh basil leaves
2 cups loosely packed fresh parsley leaves
2 cloves garlic, crushed and peeled
¼ cup plus 3 tablespoons extra virgin olive oil
3 medium zucchini or 16 ounces zucchini "noodles"
Kosher salt
Freshly ground black pepper
2 pounds large shrimp, peeled, deveined, and tails removed

1. Preheat oven to 350 degrees. Spread the nuts on a baking sheet and toast until golden, about 5 minutes. Let cool.
2. In a mini food processor or blender, combine the nuts, basil, parsley, and garlic, and pulse to make a coarse paste. With the machine running, add ¼ cup of the olive oil in a slow, steady stream until pesto is smooth. Transfer half of the pesto to a large bowl.
3. Prepare the zucchini noodles using the spiralizer (skip this step if you've bought pre-spiralized zucchini).

4. Heat a large skillet over medium-high heat. Season the shrimp thoroughly with 1 teaspoon salt and some pepper. Add 2 tablespoons olive oil to the skillet and sear the shrimp in batches until just cooked through, about 3 minutes per batch. Add the shrimp to the large bowl and toss with the pesto.

5. To the same skillet, add the remaining tablespoon of olive oil and the zucchini noodles, and season with ½ teaspoon salt and some pepper. Toss to coat the zucchini in the oil and cook until it just begins to wilt, about 2 minutes. Remove the skillet from the heat and add the remaining pesto, tossing well to coat the zucchini in the pesto. Top with half of the shrimp and serve.

About 8 grams of carbs per serving (⅛ of the shrimp plus ¼ of the zucchini noodles)

QUICK PORK AND VEGGIE CHILI

SERVES 4 PLUS LEFTOVERS

The addition of spicy chorizo and salsa makes this chili very flavorful without a long cooking time.

Use leftovers to make one of these additional recipes, available online:
- Cheesy Chili Stuffed Peppers
- Chili Quesadillas with Southwestern Slaw

Other ideas for leftovers:
- Fill an omelet with a little chili and cheese.
- Stuff chili into a baked sweet potato and top with sour cream or plain Greek yogurt.

....

2 tablespoons extra virgin olive oil
2 pounds ground pork
12 ounces fresh chorizo (or other spicy sausage), removed from the casings
Kosher salt
1 large onion, chopped
1 large bell pepper, chopped
10 ounces white or cremini mushrooms, chopped
2 medium zucchini, chopped
3 cloves garlic, chopped
2 tablespoons chili powder
1 tablespoon ground cumin

1 tablespoon paprika (or smoked paprika if you have it)
1 (28-ounce) can diced fire-roasted tomatoes
1 (16-ounce) jar spicy tomato salsa
2 cups water
Hot sauce, to taste
Grated cheddar cheese, sour cream, and chopped scallions for garnish

1. In a large pot or Dutch oven, heat the oil over medium-high heat. Add the ground pork and chorizo. Season with ½ teaspoon salt. Cook and crumble the meat until no longer pink, about 4 minutes. Add the onion, bell pepper, mushrooms, zucchini, and garlic, and cook until the vegetables begin to wilt, about 6 to 7 minutes.
2. Sprinkle the meat and vegetables with the chili powder, cumin, and paprika, and stir to coat with the spices. Add the diced tomatoes, salsa, and water. Bring to a brisk simmer over medium heat and cook until the chili has thickened and is flavorful, about 15 to 20 minutes. Season with salt and hot sauce.
3. Serve the chili topped with cheese, sour cream, and scallions.

About 18 grams of carbs per serving (1½ cups chili plus grated cheese and 1 tablespoon sour cream)

QUINOA AND ROASTED VEGETABLE BOWL WITH QUICK PEANUT SAUCE

SERVES 4 PLUS LEFTOVERS

There is a natural coating on quinoa that can be bitter, so always rinse it well in a fine strainer before cooking. If you can, leave the baking sheets in the oven while you preheat it—when you spread the vegetables on the hot baking sheets, that will start the browning process right away, ensuring a beautiful, caramelized crust.

This peanut sauce is quick to throw together and will last in the refrigerator for a week. You can use it on all kinds of cooked and raw vegetables, and it's also great on almost any cooked meat or poultry. If you don't want to make it from scratch, you can also use a jarred peanut sauce; just look at the carbs on the label to make sure it's not packed with sugar.

Use leftovers to make one of these additional recipes, available online:
- Quinoa-Crusted Chicken Fingers and One-Pan Quinoa
- Chicken Sausage Skillet with Baby Kale

Other ideas for leftovers:

- Leftover quinoa can be used in place of rice for a healthier stir-fry.
- A cup of leftover roasted vegetables would be a great addition to a frittata or an omelet.

....

3 cups chicken or vegetable broth
1½ cups quinoa, rinsed well and drained
1 large red onion, cut into chunks and separated
1 pound white mushrooms, quartered
4 tablespoons extra virgin olive oil, divided
4 teaspoons curry powder, divided
Kosher salt
Freshly ground black pepper
1 bunch medium asparagus, tough stems peeled if desired and
    asparagus cut into 2-inch pieces
2 bell peppers, any color, cut into chunks
½ cup natural peanut butter
½ cup coconut milk or hot water
Juice of 1 lime
1 tablespoon soy sauce
1 teaspoon honey or agave
1 (5-ounce) clamshell baby spinach or other baby greens

1. Preheat oven to 450 degrees.
2. Bring the broth to a boil in a small saucepan. Add the quinoa and adjust the heat to a simmer, then cover and cook 15 minutes. Remove from the heat and let sit 5 minutes, covered. Fluff with a fork.
3. In a large bowl, toss the onion and mushrooms with 2 tablespoons of the olive oil and 2 teaspoons of the curry powder. Season with salt and pepper. Spread on one of the baking sheets. Toss the asparagus and peppers in the same bowl with the remaining 2 tablespoons olive oil and 2 teaspoons curry powder. Spread on the second baking sheet.
4. Roast everything until tender and caramelized, tossing once, about 15 minutes for the mushrooms and onions and 10 minutes for the asparagus and peppers.
5. Meanwhile, in a medium bowl whisk together the peanut butter, coconut milk (or hot water), lime juice, soy sauce, and honey or agave to make a smooth, thick sauce. Add more hot water a few teaspoons at a time if the sauce is too thick. (This can also be done in a blender or food processor.)

6. To serve, divide the greens among 4 bowls and top each with ½ cup cooked quinoa. Divide all of the asparagus and peppers and half of the onions and mushrooms among the bowls. Drizzle half the peanut sauce over the four servings. Reserve the remaining mushrooms and onions, quinoa, and peanut sauce for other recipes.

About 30 grams of carbs per serving (½ cup quinoa, ⅛ mushrooms and onions, ¼ asparagus and peppers, ⅛ of the peanut sauce)

ROASTED FLANK STEAK WITH CHEESY BROCCOLI

SERVES 4 PLUS LEFTOVERS

Preheating the baking sheets in the oven is a good way to get a crispy crust on the broccoli and steak without dirtying an extra skillet on the stove.

The broccoli stems are also edible! Peel them and chop them, and you can add to the florets here, save for soups or sauces, or use in a pesto.

Use leftovers to make one of these additional recipes, available online:
- Steak and Broccoli Hash with Fried Eggs
- Quick Steak and Broccoli Fried Rice

Other ideas for leftovers:
- Chop up leftover cheesy broccoli to use in an omelet or frittata.
- For a quick stroganoff, sauté sliced onions and mushrooms in butter and add a little white wine and cream to make them saucy. Add sliced steak and warm it through. Finish with chopped parsley for color.

....

2 heads (about 2 pounds) broccoli, broken into florets
4 tablespoons extra virgin olive oil, divided
Kosher salt
Freshly ground black pepper
2 flank steaks (about 2¼ to 2½ pounds total), trimmed of excess fat
1½ tablespoons light brown sugar
1 tablespoon chili powder
½ cup finely shredded cheddar cheese

1. Preheat oven to 450 degrees. Preheat 2 large baking sheets (preferably nonstick) on the top and bottom racks of the oven.
2. Put the broccoli in a large bowl and drizzle with 2 tablespoons of the olive oil. Toss and season with ½ teaspoon salt and some pepper.

3. Rub the steaks all over with 1 tablespoon olive oil each. In a small bowl, combine the brown sugar, chili powder, 1 teaspoon salt, and some pepper. Rub the mixture all over both steaks.

4. Place a steak on each of the preheated baking sheets and roast for 5 minutes. Flip the steaks and rotate the pans between the top and bottom racks. Continue to roast the steaks until an instant-read thermometer inserted in the center of each steak registers 120 degrees for medium rare—about 5 minutes more, depending on thickness. Let the steaks rest on a cutting board while you roast the broccoli.

5. Carefully wipe the baking sheets with a paper towel. Spread the broccoli on the baking sheets and roast, tossing once about halfway through, until broccoli is tender and browned on the edges—about 10 minutes. Remove one pan of broccoli and set aside. On the other baking sheet, push the broccoli toward the middle of the pan and sprinkle with the cheese. Roast until the cheese melts, about 2 minutes.

6. Thinly slice one steak crosswise against the grain and serve with the cheesy broccoli. Reserve the other steak and the plain roasted broccoli for leftovers.

About 14 grams of carbs per serving (¼ of a flank steak plus ¼ of the cheesy broccoli)

SLOW-COOKER BBQ CHICKEN

SERVES 4 PLUS LEFTOVERS

Browning the chicken and onions is an extra step, and worth it for the depth of flavor it adds, but if you're really pressed for time, you can skip it. I like to use dark meat (such as boneless, skinless thighs) in the slow cooker as breasts tend to dry out quickly. You could also use skinless breasts, but keep them on the bone so they stay juicy, and cook them about an hour less.

Use leftovers to make one of these additional recipes, available online:
- BBQ Chicken Pizza with Cauliflower Crust
- BBQ Chicken Tostadas with Avocado and Tomato Salad

Other ideas for leftovers:
- Don't shred all of the thighs. Serve whole thighs and sauce over roasted sweet potatoes or cooked greens.

- Serve warm BBQ chicken over a scoop of quinoa (½ cup is about 20 grams of carbs) and top with avocado, tomato, red onion, and a squeeze of lime juice.

....

3 pounds boneless, skinless chicken thighs, trimmed of excess fat
1 tablespoon paprika (or smoked paprika, if you have it)
1 tablespoon mild chili powder
½ teaspoon granulated garlic
Kosher salt
Freshly ground black pepper
2 tablespoons extra virgin olive oil
2 medium onions, sliced
¼ cup tomato paste
3 tablespoons cider vinegar
3 tablespoons brown sugar
1 tablespoon Dijon mustard
2 teaspoons Worcestershire sauce
¼ cup water
1 pint prepared coleslaw, for serving

1. Season the chicken with the paprika, chili powder, granulated garlic, 1 teaspoon salt, and a generous grinding of pepper. Use your fingers to rub the spices into the chicken.
2. Heat a large skillet over medium-high heat and add the olive oil. When the oil is hot, add the chicken and brown on both sides, working in batches, about 1 minute per side. Add the chicken pieces to the slow cooker as they are browned.
3. Once all of the chicken is out of the pan, add the onions and cook over medium heat until the onions are golden on the edges, about 3 to 4 minutes. Add the onions to the slow cooker.
4. In a large liquid measuring cup, mix the tomato paste, vinegar, brown sugar, Worcestershire, and ¼ cup water. Pour over the chicken and onions. Cover and cook on high until the chicken is very tender, about 4 to 5 hours (or 6 to 7 hours on low). Shred the chicken into the sauce with 2 forks. Serve the chicken with a side of coleslaw.

About 22 grams of carbs per serving (1 cup chicken plus ½ cup slaw). The chicken has 12 grams of carbs per cup—carb count on the slaw will vary depending upon the brand, but is generally about 8 to 15 grams per ½ cup.

SOY GINGER SALMON AND SWEET POTATOES

SERVES 4 PLUS LEFTOVERS

Use leftovers to make one of these additional recipes, available online:

- Salmon Cobb Salad
- Salmon Lettuce Wraps with Broccoli Slaw

Other ideas for leftovers:

- Toss leftover flaked salmon with mayo, mustard, and herbs and seasonings of your choice to make a creamy salmon salad. Serve over greens and top with something crunchy like toasted nuts or spicy pickled vegetables.
- Mash leftover salmon with an egg, a little mustard, and some bread crumbs to make a mixture that sticks together like a meatball. Form into patties, chill, then brown in a nonstick pan—they'll only take a few minutes since the salmon is already cooked.

....

⅓ cup low-sodium soy sauce
2 tablespoons peeled, grated fresh ginger
1 tablespoon Dijon mustard
1 tablespoon agave or honey
2 tablespoons extra virgin olive oil
4 small sweet potatoes (about 4 to 5 ounces each), cut into
   1-inch chunks
1 (2-pound) skinless side of salmon
Chopped scallions, for garnish, if desired
Sesame seeds, for garnish, if desired

1. Preheat oven to 425 degrees. Line a rimmed baking sheet with foil (or use a nonstick baking sheet).
2. In a large bowl, whisk together the soy sauce, ginger, Dijon, and agave or honey. Whisk in the olive oil. Transfer half of the sauce to a small bowl. Add the sweet potatoes to the large bowl and toss well.
3. Spread the sweet potatoes on another (unlined) baking sheet and roast on the bottom rack of the oven until tender, about 20 minutes, tossing once about halfway through.
4. Meanwhile, lay the salmon on the other baking sheet, rounded side up. Brush the salmon on both sides with the remaining sauce from the small bowl. Roast on the top rack until just cooked through, about 13 to 15 minutes depending on the thickness of the salmon, brushing once with the juices about halfway through.

5. Serve half of the salmon with all of the sweet potatoes, sprinkled with scallions and sesame seeds, if desired.

About 30 grams of carbs per serving (⅛ of the salmon plus ¼ of the sweet potatoes)

SPAGHETTI SQUASH WITH MARINARA SAUCE AND ITALIAN SAUSAGE

SERVES 4, WITH LEFTOVER SAUSAGE AND MARINARA SAUCE

You can use turkey sausage if you want to lighten things up a bit. If you're a vegetarian (or just want a meatless meal), make and enjoy this dish without the sausage. You can also make this recipe with a large jar of marinara sauce if you don't have time to make the sauce—just be aware of the carb count on the label and choose one with 6 grams of carbs or less per serving.

Tip: Always buy whole canned tomatoes, then crush by hand. Canned crushed or puréed tomatoes are often lower quality or damaged tomatoes that couldn't be sold whole.

Use leftovers to make one of these additional recipes, available online:
- Open-Faced Pizza Omelet with Sausage
- Zucchini Parmesan Stacks

Other ideas for leftovers:
- Bring a couple of cups of marinara to simmer in a skillet—you can poach eggs or cook sliced boneless, skinless chicken breast or shrimp in the sauce. Sprinkle with Parmesan and briefly broil to crisp the top.
- If you have leftover squash, toss with a beaten egg and some grated Parmesan. Pan-fry in a nonstick skillet in olive oil until crisp. Serve the pancakes over spinach or baby kale and top with a little leftover marinara.

. . . .

1 medium spaghetti squash (about 3 to 3½ pounds), halved lengthwise
Kosher salt
3 tablespoons extra virgin olive oil, divided
5 links (about 1 pound) raw sweet or hot Italian sausage
1 small onion, chopped
4 large garlic cloves, peeled and thinly sliced
¼ teaspoon (or less, if using hot sausage) crushed red pepper flakes
2 (28-ounce) cans whole plum or San Marzano tomatoes, crushed
   by hand
1 cup water

3 sprigs fresh basil, plus a handful of fresh basil leaves
4 tablespoons grated Parmesan, divided

1. Preheat oven to 400 degrees. Line a roasting pan or rimmed baking sheet with foil. Season the cut halves of the squash with salt and place cut side down on the foil. Bake until tender all the way through, about 30 to 40 minutes, depending on size.

2. Meanwhile, heat a large, deep skillet or Dutch oven over medium heat. Add 2 tablespoons of the olive oil. When the oil is hot, add the sausages and brown on all sides, about 2 to 3 minutes. Push the sausages to the side and add the onion and garlic. Cook until the onion wilts, about 3 minutes. Season with 1 teaspoon salt and the red pepper flakes, and add the tomatoes and 1 cup water. Submerge the basil sprigs in the sauce, bring to a brisk simmer, and cook until sauce is flavorful and slightly thickened, about 15 to 20 minutes. Discard the basil sprigs. Tear the handful of fresh basil into the sauce and stir.

3. With a fork, scrape the squash into a large bowl (you should have about 6 cups scraped squash—if there is more, reserve for another recipe). Drizzle with the remaining olive oil and season with salt and toss. Divide among 4 pasta bowls. Top each with a sausage, ½ cup marinara sauce, and 1 tablespoon of the grated Parmesan. Reserve the remaining sausage and the rest of the marinara for other recipes.

About 16 grams of carbs per serving (1½ cups squash, 1 sausage link plus ½ cup marinara)

ACKNOWLEDGMENTS

It's hard to know where to begin, as I am exceedingly grateful and owe so much to so many people who helped me arrive at this point. Writing a book is a team sport and I have been blessed to have an amazing team around me. Each person mentioned here seemed to fit into my life at just the right moments, bringing me faith and confidence when I needed it most.

To start, I cannot express enough thanks to my editor, Alexa Stevenson. Alexa, from the moment I met you (virtually), with your assuring eyes and your awesome red lipstick, I knew I could trust you. Your guidance and support, mentorship and expertise, have shown me what excellence and dedication mean. I will never be able to thank you enough for holding my hand through this first book. I simply could not have done it without you. I was blessed in every way to be matched with you.

To my agent, Matthew Elblonk at DiFiore and Company Management, thank you. You are so deeply intelligent, not simply as a literary agent, but about people. Each time I have approached despair, you have known exactly how to guide me through. I credit you forever with making me an author. Your belief in me and my talent, against serious odds, was transformational.

For Glenn Yeffeth and the rest of the amazing people at BenBella Books, thank you for believing in my vision and standing behind me. Thank you most of all for making a long-held dream a reality.

To Catherine—my sweet sister, you will never know what your support means to me. You see me as I truly am. You never allow me to rest on what is acceptable, but push me to be better, to make my life exceptional. You are exceptional, and I credit you with this massive accomplishment.

Mom and Dad—thank you for encouraging me to chase my dreams without fear. You sent me off to study music and acting despite the odds, and that creative and free life gave me the confidence to pursue creativity throughout the rest of my life as well. That creativity has made every venture soar.

Peggy and Steve Josefsberg, my gratitude for your undying support of everything I do runs deep. You support me as your own, and have helped me in ways you will likely never know. Know you have my appreciation and love.

Joh Morris—visionary and loyal—I am grateful to have had you as an early mentor.

For Max Stubblefield and UTA, many thanks for connecting me to so many amazing people, and for taking this very small fish into your big pond.

Charles Barkley and Marc Perman—your friendship and mentorship were key as I made the leap to starting my own company. Thank you for seeing something in me and helping me see it, too.

Jennifer Hudson—my dear friend, I will forever be grateful for the day we met. You are one of this world's amazing lights! Thank you for lending your support to this book.

Dr. Oz, thank you for your advice and counsel. Your incredible intelligence and warmth have been key supports for me.

To all of my private clients—each and every one of you has inspired this book, and informed it, too. Thank you for trusting me.

My sons, Cooper and Benji, you are the reason I push myself every day. You inspire and delight me beyond words. Thank you for your unconditional love and undying support.

And finally, my dear husband, David—my partner in this life, and the love of my life. Thank you for giving me the space and confidence I needed to soar. I live to make you proud each day.

ABOUT THE AUTHOR

Liz Josefsberg is a health, wellness, and weight loss expert with over 15 years in the industry. Liz worked for 11 years as the Director of Brand Advocacy and a Leader for Weight Watchers until she started her own consulting firm as a wellness expert. Liz is likely best known for her hands-on involvement helping Oscar-winning actress and musician, Jennifer Hudson lose weight and transform her life. She also helped Jessica Simpson shed over 50 pounds of baby weight (twice!). Other celebrity clients include Charles Barkley, Katie Couric, and Amber Riley. Liz counsels both high-profile talent and everyday clients in all areas of weight loss, balance, and nutrition. She is also the author of the revolutionary *Success Handbook* (Weight Watchers) and *Find Your Fingerprint*, sold nationally in all Weight Watchers locations. Liz's work today centers on advising companies at the cutting edge of weight loss and emerging health solutions. She consults in the wearable technology sector, creates weight loss programs for forward-thinking entities, and is deeply involved in helping technology enabled weight loss and health devices come to market. Liz's perspective is derived from her own weight loss success and insatiable quest for the newest information, technology, and education available to help men and women achieve their goals with more ease in the everyday world. Liz has consulted for companies across the country, including for one of the largest fitness chains in the U.S, Life Time Fitness, Misfit Wearables, LEVL, LifeReimagined, Stash, and more. Her insights on behavior modification, consumer behavior, customer service, and the health market have made her a sought after expert in the field.